Post-Operative
RECOVERY GUIDE

Post-Operative Instructions

and Menus for Patients

of Dental Surgery

A. K. Garg, DMD

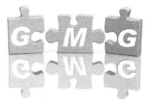

Garg Multimedia Group, inc.
1840 NE 153rd Street
North Miami Beach, FL 33162
(800) 561-3065

ISBN: 978-0-9820953-2-4

Design by Robert Mott for Robert Mott & Associates
www.RobertMottDesigns.com

Printed in the United States of America.

Contents

CHAPTER 1

Easy Post-Operative Care

Following surgery, the last thing you want to worry about is a complication due to poor post-operative care. We find that post-operative plans work best when they are conveniently woven into a patient's life, in a way that helps you concentrate on healing.

This simple-to-navigate package of information gives you top advice, treatments and habits that will expedite your healing. And we bet you will find yourself referring to it even after your recovery.

Bleeding, Pain & Swelling
Immediately After Surgery

First and foremost, after placement of dental implants, do not disturb the wound. That means avoiding any rinsing, spitting, or touching of the wound on the day of surgery. Your doctor may even advise you to avoid nose-blowing in some cases.

A small amount of bleeding, pain and swelling is perfectly normal. But, there are certain tricks to keep these post-op nuisances to a minimum.

Bleeding: Keep steady pressure over the surgical site following the procedure. Pressure helps reduce bleeding and permits the formation of a clot. Gently remove the compress after one hour. If bleeding persists, place another compress and again keep steady pressure on the area for one hour. A moistened tea bag applied to the site for 30 minutes may also help to stop bleeding. Blood or redness in the saliva is normal.

If bleeding continues, we recommend calling the office for further instructions.

It's a good idea to limit or reduce your oral activity as much as possible for several hours after surgery. Avoid any unnecessary eating, drinking and talking. These oral activities may hinder proper healing, especially in the first few hours.

Swelling: Any swelling can be minimized by applying an icepack, on the cheek or on the jaw directly, in the area of surgery. If an icepack is unavailable, simply fill a heavy plastic bag with crushed ice. Secure the end, and cover with a soft cloth to avoid skin irritation. Frozen bags of peas make wonderful icepacks and can be refrozen and used repeatedly.

Immediately following the procedure, it's advisable to apply the icepack over the affected area — 20 minutes on, and 20 minutes off — for two to four hours, to help prevent the development of excessive swelling and discomfort. Apply the ice as often as necessary, for the first 24 hours ONLY.

You may expect swelling for up to 10 days and possibly a fever of 99° to 100° F.

Pain: To minimize any discomfort from the pain, before the anesthesia wears off and feeling has returned to normal, begin taking medication as directed by your doctor.

For moderate pain, over-the-counter Tylenol or Ibuprofen comes in 200 mg tablets. Two to three tablets may be taken every three to four hours as needed to relieve the ache.

For severe pain, the prescribed medication should be taken as directed. Take the prescribed narcotic medication if you experience significant pain.

If anti-inflammatory medication was prescribed, begin taking the medication with food immediately after the procedure and continue as directed.

If you were not prescribed any anti-inflammatory medication and you don't have a known allergy to Aspirin or Ibuprofen (Motrin), you can take 600 mg of Ibuprofen (Motrin) every six hours to control mild to moderate pain. *Note: Do not take any of the above medications if you are allergic, or have been instructed by your doctor not to take it.*

Prescribed antibiotics to help prevent infection are usually started an hour or two prior to implant surgery, and continued for about a week afterward.

Cold, then warm: Remember, in terms of compresses and foods, administer cold items for the first 24 hours and then warm afterward.

Ongoing Oral Hygiene

Good oral hygiene is essential to good healing. This includes warm salt water rinses (a teaspoon of salt in a cup of warm water) at least four to five times a day. (What until 24 hours after surgery to start the rinses to minimize chance of disturbing the blood clot.) Repeat after every meal or snack for seven days. Rinsing is important because it removes food particles and debris and thus helps promote healing.

You can also brush your tongue with a dry toothbrush to keep bacteria growth down, but be careful not to touch the surgical site. Resume your regular tooth brushing after two days, but still avoid disturbing the surgical area.

Diet

Eating might seem like the last thing on your mind after dental surgery, but it's still important to nourish your body. Drink plenty of fluids. Avoid hot liquids or food. Soft, cool food and liquids should be consumed on the day of surgery, returning to a normal diet over the course of two weeks.

> **WARNING: for two weeks after surgery do not eat or drink:**
> - Spicy foods
> - Acidic juices (orange, grapefruit, etc.)
> - Chips
> - Popcorn
> - Carbonated drinks

Maintain proper diet: Have your meals at the usual time. Eat soft, nutritious foods, and hydrate your mouth regularly with liquids, during meals and in between. However, always be careful not to disturb the blood clot. Add solid foods to your diet as per the schedule in the upcoming Menu section.

Wearing Your Prosthesis

Partial or full dentures should not be used immediately after surgery, and for at least 10 days, unless allowed by your doctor.

Activity

It's wise to keep physical activities to a minimum immediately following surgery. Rest up and heal; otherwise you could be setting your recovery back by a few days. If you engage in vigorous exercise, throbbing or bleeding at the surgical site may occur. If this happens, you should discontinue exercising. Keep in mind that you are probably not taking in the normal amount of calories for normal exercise. This may weaken you and further limit your ability.

If you should have any problems such as excessive bleeding, pain, or difficulty in opening your mouth, call the office immediately for further instructions, assistance, or additional treatment.

Remember your follow-up visit: You will be scheduled to return for a post-operative visit to make certain healing is progressing satisfactorily. While you wait for that appointment, maintain a healthful diet, observe the basic rules for proper oral hygiene, and call the office if you have any questions or concerns.

Post-Op Care Recap

Here are the top 10 tips for care after surgery:

1. **Don't Touch!** Keep fingers and tongue away from surgical area.

2. **Cool It!** Use ice packs on surgical area (side of face) for the first 12 hours; apply ice 20 minutes on, 20 minutes off. Bags of frozen peas work quite well for this.

3. **Still Hurts?** For mild discomfort, take Tylenol or Ibuprofen every three to four hours.

4. **In Pain?** For severe pain, please use the prescription medication for pain given to you.

5. **Hydrate Yourself.** Drink plenty of fluids. Do not use a straw.

6. **Chew Gum.** If the muscles of the jaw become stiff, chewing gum at intervals will help relax the muscles. The use of warm, moist heat on the outside of your face beginning on the second day after surgery will further help with relaxation of the muscle.

7. **Eat Soft Foods.** Diet may consist of soft foods, which can be easily chewed and swallowed. Recommended foods and recipes are provided in the Menu section. No seeds, nuts, rice, or popcorn!

8. **Blood?** A certain amount of bleeding can be expected following surgery. Bleeding is controlled by applying pressure to the surgical area for 90 minutes. Then you may eat or drink. If bleeding persists, a moist tea bag should be held firmly on the area of bleeding for one hour straight.

9. **No Smoking, Please!** Do not smoke for at least five days after surgery.

10. **Drugs?** If you are on other medications, be sure to discuss this with your doctor or pharmacist to minimize adverse drug interactions. Do start taking a multi-vitamin daily, however, if you are not already doing so.

CHAPTER 2

The First 24 Hours

A fter surgery, some people find it difficult to eat or enjoy their food. This reluctance to sit down at meal times, plus an inability to consume normal, solid food, is especially true after dental surgery.

It's not difficult to see why: too much chewing, slurping or sucking can aggravate the treated area, resulting in discomfort and even pain. It also can potentially re-open the area, causing bleeding or infection that will delay healing or cause problems with the surgery if the area is disturbed too much. However, despite any fears or lack of appetite, it's vital that you continue to eat, as nutrients provide energy and facilitate your healing process on the road to recovery.

Many patients ask, "What types of food are best?" "What sort of meals should be avoided?" In general, the rule of thumb is: no spicy foods, chips, popcorn, acidic juices, or carbonated drinks. But we prefer to go a step further and provide a series of menu suggestions that are both inventive and nutritious for the body.

Thus, we've compiled a list of appropriate and delicious menus, suitable for each stage of your two-week recovery, beginning from the first 24 hours, to days 2 to 5, and finally days 5 to 14. Each section includes several drink recipes, main courses and a few sweet choices.

Before commencing with the recipes, there is also a quick reference list, which includes more general suggestions on what is good to eat during a specific period. Those noted with a "star" (*) indicate that the recipe will follow.

Whether you or a friend or family member will be donning the chef's hat, we hope you enjoy a comfortable and tasty dining experience. Bon appetit!

The day of your surgery and for the first 24 hours following, it's a good idea to give your teeth a bit of a break. For this reason, cold soups, smoothies, jello/puddings, and cold drinks should be your main dietary intake. And remember, refrain from using a straw, because the sucking action can cause excess strain, move the newly formed blood clot, and delay your ultimate recovery.

Suggestions for Day 1

BEVERAGES:

Banana-Mango Shake *

Blackberry-Orange Cooler *

Chocolate Banana Smoothie *

Coffee Granita *

Iced Tea

Milk

Milk Shake (no straws allowed)

Nutritional Supplement Drink (e.g., Slim•Fast, Carnation Instant
  Breakfast, Ensure)

Strawberry-Blueberry Smoothie *

Water

MAINS:

Cold Pasta

French Ratatouille Soup *

Orange-Carrot Soup *

Gazpacho Soup *

Mango-Melon Soup *

Mashed Potatoes

Mexican Avocado Soup *

Apple and Potato Soup *

Tomato Soup *

Ukrainian Lenten Borscht *

DESSERTS:

Applesauce *

Cold Pudding

Jell-O Desserts

Lush Chocolate Mousse *

Yogurt or Kefir

BEVERAGES

Banana-Mango Shake

South Florida is said to have a cuisine all its own. The diversity of its people also combines a wide variety of flavors that stimulate the palate and the imagination, earning them the title of "Floribbean." Some of the things that give SoFla its identity are its abundance of fresh, tropical fruit. Bananas are a natural source of potassium, which makes them popular with athletes and those with high blood pressure. But they also help replace electrolytes, the charges needed to power the body and maintain fluid balance. The enzymes inside mango, such as magneferin, katechol oxidase and lactase, clean the bowels and also help the body maintain resistance to fight germs. Aside from all of that, they taste great together. We strongly recommend making this shake fresh at home.

INGREDIENTS:

- ½ banana
- 1 cup mango, peeled, pitted and chopped
- ½ cup plain yogurt
- 1 cup of ice cubes
- non-acidic juice (e.g., apple) or milk as needed

DIRECTIONS:

Place all ingredients in a blender and puree until smooth. Add juice or milk gradually until shake is the desired consistency/thickness.

Coffee Granita

In Italy, people enjoy a wide variety of juicy and tasty beverages in an icy form called a "granita." During hot summers, they use espresso to create espresso granitas. These icy frozen mixtures first appeared in Europe around the 17th century. They are so simple, you'll want them all year. Granitas are the perfect morning pick-me-up.

INGREDIENTS:

- Espresso, pre-brewed and cooled (sweeten if desired)

DIRECTIONS:

Use a 9x13 inch metal or glass pan. Pour espresso into the pan and freeze for 20 minutes. Use a whisk to rake the frozen edges toward the center and place in freezer again. Repeat raking into the center and freezing every 20 minutes until frozen through, about five hours. Cover and keep frozen. Use a fork to stir the granita again just before serving, and mold with an ice-cream scoop.

Blackberry-Orange Cooler

Throughout the world and throughout history, the citrus fruit has been a symbol of health and beauty. The very wealthy presented citrus to each other as precious gifts, and citrus is still a primary ingredient in perfume and aromatherapy. Blackberries help combat nausea and also are high in Vitamin E, which promotes healing. Here is a recipe that incorporates both, for your enjoyment.

INGREDIENTS:

- 4 blackberries
- ½ cup plain yogurt
- ½ cup orange juice
- sugar or sweetener to taste (Splenda does not raise the glycemic index)
- 1 scoop vanilla whey protein powder (optional)

(Continued on next page.)

DIRECTIONS:

Place all ingredients in the blender and blend at high speed for one minute, or until blackberries are liquefied. Strain to eliminate all seeds. Pour into a large glass, and drink!

Chocolate Banana Smoothie

This recipe is for your inner child and your outer body. Flaxseed oil is full of omega-3, a natural antioxidant. It also helps prevent constipation, a common post-op complaint due to antibiotics and pain medication. Pamper yourself with the flavors you craved when you were a kid and the ingredients you need as an adult.

INGREDIENTS:

- 1 tsp. cocoa powder
- ½ ripe banana
- ½ cup plain yogurt
- 1 tsp. of sugar, or 1 packet sweetener
- ½ cup water
- 1-2 large ice cubes
- 1 tsp. flaxseed oil (if available)
- 1 scoop whey protein powder (optional)

DIRECTIONS:

Combine all ingredients in a blender and blend at high speed for 30 seconds. Add 1 or 2 large ice cubes and blend for another 30 seconds, or until smooth. Enjoy.

Strawberry-Blueberry Smoothie

Some of you might already know that the blueberry has a compound that inhibits the production of precancerous cells by literally deflating them. It is called pterostilbene. Their midnight-blue coloration has a purpose other than attractiveness. It's caused by polyphenol pigments called anthocyanins, which come from a potent family of antioxidants that prevent cancer in all three phases: initiation, promotion and proliferation. And because you are also trying to stay healthy during your recovery, blueberries are ideal because they have an anti-adhesion effect which prevents common urinary tract infections and E. coli from invading you. It's just plain bananas not to eat these mini miracle-workers because they are so easy to prepare: no peeling, pitting, coring, or cutting.

INGREDIENTS:

- ½ cup strawberries
- ½ cup blueberries
- ¾ cup apple juice
- ½ cup ice
- 1 scoop of plain lowfat yogurt (optional)

DIRECTIONS:

Blend together the strawberries and blueberries with a splash of apple juice until liquefied. Then add in the remainder of the apple juice, ice, and optional plain lowfat yogurt, blending until nice and smooth.

MAIN COURSES
French Ratatouille Soup

If cooking is not your strength, then this recipe might intrigue you for many reasons. First, you can create something from nothing (or leftovers). Second, the wide range of vitamins and nutrients found in this soup can help promote and regulate various chemical processes within your body. And third, this classic Provençal dish is good hot, cold or pureed.

INGREDIENTS:

- 2 tbsp. olive oil
- 1 large onion, chopped
- 1 tsp. garlic, chopped
- 1 medium zucchini, chopped
- 1 small eggplant, chopped
- 1 bell pepper, chopped (any color)
- 2 lbs. fresh or canned tomatoes, peeled and chopped
- 1 tsp. fresh thyme, minced (or ¼ teaspoon dried)
- 2 cups vegetable or chicken stock
- pinch of cayenne pepper
- 1 tsp. salt (ideally, sea salt, that great *sel de mer* from France)
- ⅛ tsp. freshly ground black pepper
- 2 tbsp. fresh basil, sliced fine, for garnish
- Balsamic vinegar, for garnish

DIRECTIONS:

Heat the olive oil in a large saucepan or Dutch oven. Sauté the onion and garlic until soft, three to four minutes, over medium heat. Add the chopped eggplant, zucchini and pepper, sautéing for color, and to soften the vegetables, approximately five minutes, stirring occasionally. Gradually stir in the tomatoes and their juices, followed by the spices and vegetable stock. Bring the liquid to a boil. Then reduce the heat and simmer for 15–20 minutes.

(Continued on next page.)

You can serve the soup warm and chunky or as a puree, either warm or cold. If opting for the puree, ladle the solids into the blender first, and gradually add the broth, until you reach the desired consistency. In either case, garnish with a little balsamic vinegar in each bowl and sprinkle with fresh basil. If eaten during the first 24 hours after surgery, it should be eaten chilled.

Orange-Carrot Soup

Carrots are high in vitamins A, B and C, and contain beta carotene, which helps prevent heart disease and several different types of cancers, including oral cancer.

INGREDIENTS:

- 2 tbsp. peanut oil
- 1 lb. carrots, coarsely chopped
- ¾ cup sliced leeks, white part only
- 1 tbsp. fresh ginger root, peeled and minced
- 3 cups chicken or vegetable stock
- 1½ cups fresh squeezed orange juice
- salt, to taste
- 2 tbsp. sliced leeks, separated into circles, for garnish

DIRECTIONS:

Heat the oil in a large saucepan. Once hot, sauté the carrots, leeks and ginger until they are soft. Add stock and bring to a boil. Reduce heat and simmer, covered, for about 20-30 minutes, until vegetables are well-cooked. Purée the mixture, beginning with the solids. Once smooth, return to the soup to the saucepan. Stir in the orange juice and season to taste with salt. (Note that cold soups often require additional salt to help bring out the flavors.) Refrigerate and chill. When cool, garnish bowls with finely-sliced leek circles.

Gazpacho Soup

Gazpacho soup is the original "V8." All good comfort food is usually derived from "poor people food," and gazpacho soup is no different, being the food that farm workers enjoyed in Andalusia, Spain. Gazpacho is a sultry mix of everyday garden vegetables, and, if you've never had a cold soup before, this rich burst of flavors will make you a convert. Although there are many regional and modern versions of this soup, it's traditionally made with ripe tomatoes, bell peppers, cucumbers, and garlic. But the main reason we've included it here is because all the ingredients reduce inflammation and tissue damage, prevent disease and cell damage, and relieve stress!

INGREDIENTS:

- 4 cups tomato juice
- 1 onion, minced
- 1 green bell pepper, minced
- 1 cucumber, chopped
- 2 cups chopped tomatoes
- 2 green onions, chopped
- 1 clove garlic, minced
- 3 tbsp. fresh lemon juice
- 2 tbsp. red wine vinegar
- 1 tsp. dried tarragon
- 1 tsp. dried basil
- ¼ cup chopped fresh parsley
- 1 tsp. white sugar
- salt and pepper, to taste

DIRECTIONS:

In a blender, combine all ingredients, except salt and pepper. Pulse until well-combined but still slightly chunky. Taste the soup, adding seasoning (salt and pepper) as needed. Chill at least two hours before serving.

Mango-Melon Soup

As we said before, mangos are a wonderful part of tropical cuisine and help purify the intestinal tract. This soup is head and shoulders above the rest to stabilize a tender tummy while recovering from surgery.

INGREDIENTS:

- 2 mangoes, peeled, pitted, and chopped
- 2 cups cantaloupe, peeled, seeded, and chopped
- 2 tbsp. fresh mint, minced
- 2 tbsp. fresh lemon juice
- 1 tbsp. confectioner's sugar
- ¼ cup dry white wine
- 2 tbsp. plain yogurt
- 2 tsp. edible flowers (if available), for garnish
- 2 tsp. small mint leaves, for garnish

DIRECTIONS:

Combine all ingredients in a blender and puree. Chill for several hours. When cool, serve in glass bowls and garnish with small mint leaves, or edible flowers if available. If you'd like to serve the soup immediately, begin with the fruit having already been chilled in the refrigerator, then add a handful of ice cubes into the blender while pureeing.

Mexican Avocado Soup

For many years it's been thought that avocados were unhealthy because they contained lots of fat. Now we know those reports were only partially true: avocados are high in fat — "good fat" — the monounsaturated kind. Avocados actually will lower your cholesterol. In fact, they are extremely nutritious and contribute nearly 20 vitamins, minerals and beneficial plant compounds to your diet. Always with your health in mind, try this delicious all-season treat with a south-of-the-border twist. Serve cold.

INGREDIENTS:
- 4 cups vegetable or chicken stock
- 1 cup heavy cream, or half and half
- 1 chili pepper, as hot as you dare (from banana to habanero)
- 1 garlic clove
- 2 avocados
- salt and white pepper
- 2 tbsp. cilantro, finely chopped, for garnish
- ¼ cup crisp, fried tortillas, for garnish

DIRECTIONS:

In a saucepan, heat the stock and cream, and keep the temperature steady at a simmer. Puree the chili pepper and garlic in a blender, then add the avocado. When ready to serve, gradually add the hot stock mixture and blend until smooth. Season to taste and either serve immediately with cilantro and chips on the side, or refrigerate to make a cold soup. Note that avocados turn bitter when heated, so be careful not to add liquid that is too hot.

Apple and Potato Soup

One of the common problems that people suffer after surgery is constipation. This delicious and unique soup will put some much-needed fiber back in your body to get it moving in the right direction, as well as some vitamin C.

INGREDIENTS:

- 4 tbsp. butter
- 2 leeks (white part), sliced
- 5 cups tart apples (e.g. Granny Smith), peeled, cored, and chopped
- 6 cups chicken stock
- 2 cups potatoes, peeled and chopped
- 1 cup heavy cream, or half and half
- 2 tsp. Calvados (or apple brandy)
- ⅛ teaspoon cinnamon
- salt and white pepper, to taste
- 2 apples, peeled, cored, diced, for garnish
- 2 tbsp. butter, for garnish

DIRECTIONS:

In a large saucepan, melt the butter. Sauté the leeks over medium heat, covered, for three to four minutes. Toss in the apples and cook, uncovered, for about five minutes, coating them well with the butter. Pour in the stock, add the potatoes, and bring the mixture to a boil. Reduce heat and simmer for 45 minutes. When the apples and potatoes are soft, puree the mixture in a blender—solids first—until smooth. Return the puree to the saucepan, and slowly stir in the cream, Calvados and cinnamon. Season to taste. In a separate pan, sauté the diced apple in two tablespoons of butter until soft, for about 5 minutes. Remove from heat and drain on a paper towel until ready to serve. Refrigerate if you are going to serve cold (in which case you will want to over-season a bit). When ready to serve, top the soup with the diced apple garnish.

Tomato Soup

Tomatoes are an excellent source of vitamin C, which boosts your immune system.

INGREDIENTS:

- 3 pounds fresh or canned tomatoes, peeled, seeded, and chopped
- 1 onion, chopped
- 1 clove garlic, chopped
- 1 bay leaf
- several sprigs of thyme (or ¼ teaspoon dried)
- 1 tbsp. olive oil
- ½ tsp. brown sugar
- pinch of nutmeg
- pinch of paprika
- 1 egg yolk
- 2 tbsp. crème fraîche, or sour cream
- salt and pepper, to taste
- ¼ cup freshly grated Parmesan cheese, for garnish
- 2 tbsp. thinly sliced basil, for garnish

DIRECTIONS:

In a large saucepan, stir together all the ingredients except the egg yolk and crème fraiche. Bring the mixture to a boil and cook on medium heat for 40 minutes. Remove the bay leaf and sprigs of thyme. Turn heat to high and bring the soup to a boil for a minute or two.

Place soup in a blender and puree until smooth. Return soup to the pan and reheat at a simmer. Right before serving, beat the egg yolk with the crème fraîche. Whisk the egg-crème fraîche mixture into the pot and cook, stirring, on low heat until the soup thickens. When ready to serve, set out the soup plates (warming them is nice), ladle in the soup and top with Parmesan and slivers of basil leaf. You also can serve the soup cold with a splash of cream in each bowl.

Hot Borscht (Ukrainian Lenten Borscht)

If you live in or near any major U.S. city, you've probably run into at least one Ukrainian restaurant or family (even better), who serve borscht. This beet-based stew is distinctive for its reddish pink color and amazing array of vegetables. No other stew in the world can compare to its nutritional value. This is the stew that fed armies who fought in World Wars I and II, trudging through miles of snow and ice. It can surely get you back on your feet, too. The betacyanin pigment that gives beets their color is also a powerful cancer-fighting antioxidant!

INGREDIENTS:

- ½ ounce dried porcini (bolete) mushrooms, soaked in hot water for 30 minutes, then julienned, reserving the liquid
- 10 cups water
- 1 carrot, grated
- salt and black pepper, to taste
- 1 tbsp. vegetable oil, using more as needed
- 2 medium red beets, cut into a julienne
- 1 large onion, diced fine
- 2 carrots, cut into a julienne
- 3 medium potatoes, peeled and sliced
- 1 bay leaf
- ½ head of a medium-sized cabbage, sliced finely
- 2 7-ounce tins of fish fillets in tomato sauce
- 3 tbsp. tomato paste
- up to 2 tbsp. apple cider vinegar
- 2 cloves puréed garlic, for garnish
- 2 tbsp. chopped dill, for garnish

(Continued on next page.)

DIRECTIONS:

In a large pot, bring the water and mushroom-soaking liquid to a boil. Reduce the heat, and stir in carrots, mushrooms, and salt, keeping everything at a simmer. In a frying pan, heat the oil at a low heat. Toss in the julienned beets, and let them sweat for 35 minutes. Then, add them into the simmering soup liquid. In the same frying pan, add a little more oil; toss in the onion and carrots, and soften, letting them sweat for 10 minutes. Again, add them into the soup. Then, toss the sliced potatoes, bay leaf, and pepper into the soup and cook until the potatoes are tender. At that point, add in the cabbage, cooking until done to your preference (either crunchy or soft). Finally, remove the bay leaf and add the tomato paste and fish, broken into medium chunks with a fork. Add salt and pepper as necessary. The soup should have a sour note, which you can strengthen with as much as two tablespoons of vinegar. When ready to serve, stir in the pureed garlic and chopped dill. The soup also may be chilled and served cold.

DESSERTS

Applesauce

The Bible takes much credit for the popularity of the apple, but sadly, hieroglyphics on the walls of the ancient tombs of Ramses II show that apples have been around even longer. Apples, and subsequently, applesauce, actually trace their ancestry to the days of prehistoric man. Stone tablets depict ancient residents of what is now Switzerland cooking apples. Later, ancient Greeks created recipes and elixirs that contained apples, as well as a simple applesauce. No need to fix what is not broken, so enjoy this ancient dish filled with bacteria-killing properties. Our version omits the use of sugar, so you can maximize the benefits.

INGREDIENTS:

- 3 sweet apples, peeled, cored and quartered
- zest of ½ lemon
- 1½ tsp. lemon juice
- ½ tsp. cinnamon
- ¼ cup of water

DIRECTIONS:

Combine all ingredients in a saucepan and bring to a boil. Reduce heat, cover and simmer for 15 minutes, or until apples are very soft. Mash with a fork, and season cinnamon if needed. Chill and enjoy!

Lush Chocolate Mousse

By now you should know that dark, unsweetened chocolate is great for lowering blood pressure. But did you also know that chocolate helps improve your mood? Indulge in this sumptuous dessert while you recover. You don't need to feel guilty anymore.

INGREDIENTS:

- 1½ cups of whipping cream
- 8 ounces of unsweetened dark chocolate, melted
- 2 tbsp. sugar
- ½ tsp. vanilla

DIRECTIONS:

In a saucepan, warm half of the whipping cream (¾ cup) and remove from heat. Add sugar and vanilla to the melted chocolate, then combine chocolate mixture with the heated cream. In a separate bowl, whip remaining cream until it has soft peaks. At that point, slowly fold it into the chocolate mixture. Divide into small bowls or glasses and chill until set.

BEVERAGES:

Apple Cider *

Banana-Peanut Butter Shake *

Coffee

Milk

Nutritional Supplement drink (eg: Slim•Fast, Carnation Instant
  Breakfast, Ensure)

Ovaltine Chocolate Malt

Peach Iced Tea *

Rich Hot Chocolate *

Tea – Green, Black or Herbal

Water

BREAKFAST:

Broccoli Omelette *

French Toast *

Hot Oatmeal *

Pancakes *

Scrambled Eggs

Soft Cereals

Waffles

BREADS:

Honey/Wheat Bread (with crusts broken off)

Rolls

Soft Brown Bread

White Bread

SOUPS:

Bortolli Bean Soup *

Butternut Squash Soup *

Cheesy Potato and Corn Chowder *

Chicken Tortilla Soup *

Chickpea Noodle Soup *

San Francisco Cioppino *

Creamed Broccoli and Mushroom Soup *

Ham and Potato Soup *

Indian Mulligatawny Soup *

Italian Sausage Soup *

Lentil Soup *

Harira (Moroccan Lamb Soup) *

Quick and Easy Chicken Noodle Soup *

Split Pea Soup *

Taco Soup *

Texas Corn Chowder *

Tortilla and Bean Soup *

Vegetable Soup *

Vegetarian Split Pea Soup *

LUNCH/DINNER:

Chicken Pesto Pasta*

Chickpea Hot Pot Recipe *

Fish Fillets (steamed or baked)

Fish in Foil *

Frittata *

Grilled Cheese Sandwich

Lamb and Winter Vegetable Stew *

Macaroni and Cheese

Meatloaf

Mediterranean Fish Stew *

Okra Stew with Shrimp *

Orzo Shrimp Stew *

Quiche *

Rajasthani "Buttermilk" Curry *

Warm Pasta Dishes

DESSERTS:

Apple Rhubarb Crumble *

Bread and Butter Pudding *

Crème Brulée

Cold Puddings

Fruit with Warm Custard

Jell-O Desserts

Rice Pudding

Strawberry Parfait *

Very Berry Pie *

Yogurt or Kefir

BEVERAGES

Apple Cider

Long touted by ancient Egyptians to be an elixir of eternal youth, apple cider is indeed a natural multi-vitamin and mineral treasure trove. Even Hippocrates — the father of medicine — acknowledged the vast healing properties of apple cider.

INGREDIENTS:

- 2 cups apple juice
- 1 cinnamon stick, 2 inches
- 3 cloves (whole)
- 2 tbsp. orange peel
- sugar, if desired

DIRECTIONS:

Place all ingredients in a saucepan and bring to a simmer. Cover and continue to simmer for 15–20 minutes. Taste and add sugar if desired. Strain and serve warm.

Banana-Peanut Butter Shake

Peanut butter is rich in protein, giving this shake an energy boost. It is also known to help protect against heart disease.

INGREDIENTS:

- 1 cup milk
- 1 tbsp. creamy peanut butter
- ½ banana
- 1 scoop protein powder (optional)

DIRECTIONS:

Place all ingredients in a blender and puree until smooth. Enjoy!

Peach Iced Tea

Tea is known for its antioxidants and healing properties, while peaches, a source of natural sugars, also contain vitamins A and C. You can even add a bit of peach pureé to create a mock Bellini. This beverage is a great twist on an old favorite.

INGREDIENTS:

- 3 cups water
- 3 tea bags
- 3 tbsp. sugar
- 1 cinnamon stick, 2 inches
- 1 cup peach nectar
- 1 peach, sliced in thin wedges

DIRECTIONS:

Boil the water, and make tea. Once steeped to your preference, three to five minutes, remove tea bags. Add sugar and cinnamon while liquid is still warm, and stir to dissolve. Mix in peach juice and peach slices. Chill in the fridge before serving over ice.

Rich Hot Chocolate

In the ancient Maya culture, a cacao beverage was consumed for medicinal properties. Today we have returned to this use for chocolate's antioxidant properties and ability to lower blood pressure. The best way to enjoy chocolate for its benefits and prevent a high calorie intake is to keep it pure. Use only the finest unsweetened dark chocolate.

INGREDIENTS:

- 1½ cups fat-free milk
- 3 tbsp. turbinado sugar
- 3 ounces unsweetened dark, 70% cacao chocolate, finely chopped

DIRECTIONS:

Heat the milk and sugar together until it almost boils. Reduce heat and add in chocolate, gently stirring until melted. Serve warm. For a real treat, try topping it with whipped cream.

BREAKFAST

Broccoli Omelette

Everyone now knows broccoli's nutritive power extends beyond just multi-vitamins and antioxidants. It also contains enough calcium to supplement the diets of those who do not consume dairy products. However, are you an expert at selecting broccoli? Choose only the darkest greens and the thinnest stalks, and go for organic. Color is key: never choose yellow.

INGREDIENTS:

- 1 tbsp. vegetable oil
- 3 eggs
- dash of salt and pepper
- ⅓ cup cooked broccoli, small pieces
- ½ cup cheddar cheese, shredded

DIRECTIONS:

Warm a frying pan on medium heat and add the oil. In a bowl, beat eggs, salt and pepper together, then add the mixture to the hot pan. Turn the temperature to medium-low and cook the egg. Once the top side has set (looks mainly firm), add the cheese and broccoli to one-half of the top side of the omelette. Fold the egg in half, covering the cheese and broccoli. Cook for two to four more minutes, until cheese has melted.

French Toast

From a way to use stale bread to a full-fledged, high-end brunch item,
French toast has come a long way. Best made with thick-sliced fresh bread
and dusted with powdered sugar, our whole-wheat recipe also will give you
some much-needed fiber to keep you regular after surgery.

INGREDIENTS:

- 2 tbsp. vegetable oil
- 1 egg
- 1¼ cups milk
- 1 tsp. ground cinnamon
- dash of salt
- 4 pieces of whole-wheat bread
- maple syrup (optional)
- jam (optional)

DIRECTIONS:

Place a frying pan on medium heat and add the oil. In a wide bowl,
beat together the egg, milk, cinnamon and salt. Take a piece of bread
and dip both sides into the egg mixture. Then, place it in the pan
to cook, three to four minutes a side, or until golden brown. Repeat
with all slices. Depending on the size of your pan, you should be able
to cook multiple slices at the same time. Serve topped with maple
syrup, jam or fresh fruit.

Hot Oatmeal

In 1997, oatmeal became the first whole food to bear a "claim" label approved by the FDA. This is one of those little labels that claim the food has a property that does something good for your body. Your grandmother was right: oatmeal may reduce the risk of heart disease. Try it mixed with raisins and brown sugar so you can also remember how good her cookies were.

INGREDIENTS:
- ½ cup small, quick-cooking oats
- 1 cup water
- ¼ cup raisins
- 2 tbsp. brown sugar
- 2 tbsp. milk

DIRECTIONS:
Place oats and water into a large microwaveable bowl. Cook on high for 1½ to 2½ minutes, until oats are soft and cooked. Stir in raisins and top with brown sugar. Once the sugar has "melted," finish with milk and serve.

Pancakes

INGREDIENTS:

- 2 cups flour
- ½ tsp. salt
- 3 tbsp. sugar
- 1 tbsp. baking powder
- ½ cup blueberries
- 2 eggs
- 1¼ cups milk
- 1 tbsp. melted butter

DIRECTIONS:

Combine the dry ingredients and stir together. Add in and coat the blueberries. In a separate bowl, mix the wet ingredients, beating the eggs slightly. Combine both dry and wet ingredients together, just until mixed. (They don't need to be smooth.) Spoon the batter in small portions (¼ cup of the mixture) onto a hot, oiled frying pan, on low-medium heat. When the pancakes have "bubbles"on the top, the pancake is ready to flip. The other side will only need two to three minutes. Should your pancake be overcooked on the underside, before the bubbles appear, turn down the heat for the next batch. Serve with maple syrup, fresh fruit or simply butter.

SOUPS

Borlotti Bean Soup

Italian Borlotti beans, also known as "tongues of fire," are not like Great Northern white beans. They are creamier and heavier. It's really worth buying them at an Italian goods store for the real deal. Borlotti are an excellent source of fiber for a healthy digestive system, and a source of protein that is low in fat.

INGREDIENTS:

- 1 lb. Borlotti beans
- 8 cups water
- 15 cloves of garlic, peeled and trimmed
- 2 large shallots (or 1 white onion), sliced into thin crescents
- 2–3 dried smoked chilis (serrano pepper if available)
- 2 tsp. fine sea salt, plus additional for seasoning
- a drizzle of extra virgin olive oil
- a small handful of cilantro, chopped
- ½ cup Parmesan, grated (optional)

DIRECTIONS:

Give the beans a thorough rinse, then soak them overnight in a large pot of water, covered with a few extra inches of liquid. When you are ready to use the beans, drain and rinse them again before using. Preheat oven to 350° , with the racks near the bottom. Put the beans, water, garlic, shallots, and peppers in an oven-proof pot, preferably one with an oven-proof lid. Place the pot on a rimmed baking sheet (in case of accidental overflow), and cook in the oven for two hours, or until beans are nice and tender. After the first hour, check every 20 minutes. When the beans are done, remove from the oven and season generously with salt. Stir, taste, and season to your liking. Let the soup rest on the stovetop, covered, for 10 minutes, allowing the beans time to absorb the seasoned broth. Taste and adjust seasoning once again, finally drizzling with the olive oil. To serve, first ladle a generous scoop of beans into each bowl, followed by the broth, covering the beans. Sprinkle with fresh cilantro and grated cheese.

Butternut Squash Soup

Many of you may enjoy these delicious gourds in the winter, but did you know that they contain carotenes that have antioxidants, which help reduce the risk for many types of cancer, including oral cancer? Squash is good for you at any time of year!

INGREDIENTS:

- 2 tbsp. butter
- 1 small onion, chopped
- 1 stalk celery, chopped
- 1 medium carrot, chopped
- 2 medium potatoes, cubed
- 1 medium butternut squash, peeled, seeded and cubed
- 4 cups of chicken stock
- salt and freshly ground black pepper, to taste

DIRECTIONS:

Melt the butter in a large pot and cook the onion, celery, carrot for about five minutes, or until lightly browned. Add the potatoes and squash to the pot. Pour in just enough chicken stock to cover the vegetables, and bring to a boil. Reduce heat to low and simmer 40 minutes, covered, or until all vegetables are tender. Transfer the soup to a blender and puree until smooth. Return to the pot and add additional stock to attain desired consistency. Season with salt and pepper.

Cheesy Potato and Corn Chowder

INGREDIENTS:

- 2 tbsp. margarine
- 1 cup celery, chopped
- 1 cup onion, chopped
- 4 cups chicken broth
- 3 cups potatoes, peeled and cubed
- 1 can whole kernel corn (15 ounces)
- ½ cup diced green pepper.
- 1 pkg. country style gravy mix (2.5 ounce)
- 2 cups milk
- 1 cup shredded cheese

DIRECTIONS:

In large saucepan, melt margarine over medium heat. Add celery and onion; cook, stirring occasionally until tender, about five minutes. Add chicken broth and bring to a boil. Reduce the heat to low and add potatoes, cooking 20–25 minutes or until potatoes are soft.

Stir in corn and peppers, and return to a boil. At this point, dissolve gravy mix into the milk, before adding to the boiling mixture. Again, reduce the heat and add the cheese, cooking until melted. Stir everything together before serving.

Chicken Tortilla Soup

Tortillas, a Mexican flatbread made with ground maize, have experienced a meteoric rise in popularity that has everyone craving wraps. The fresher you can get them, the better they are for your health. When you find a nice Mexican restaurant you can trust, ask if you can buy them in bulk, and then freeze them so you can use whatever you need.

Lemon juice brightens the flavors in this gorgeous chicken, corn and salsa soup. On another note, cumin is a fantastic source of iron and calcium.

INGREDIENTS:

- 2 skinless, boneless chicken breasts
- ½ tsp. olive oil
- ½ tsp. garlic, minced
- ¼ tsp. ground cumin
- 4 cups chicken broth
- 1 cup frozen corn kernels
- 1 cup onion, chopped
- ½ tsp. chili powder
- 1 tbsp. lemon juice
- 1 cup chunky salsa
- 1 cup corn tortilla chips
- ½ cup Monterey Jack cheese, shredded (optional)

DIRECTIONS:

First, in a large pot over medium heat, saute the chicken in the oil for five minutes. Add the garlic and cumin and mix well. Then add the broth, corn, onion, chili powder, lemon juice, and salsa. Reduce heat to low and simmer for about 20-30 minutes. Before serving, break up some tortilla chips in the individual bowls. Then pour soup over the chips; top with the shredded cheese and a dollop of sour cream. Garnish with tortilla chips, grated cheese and a dollop of sour cream.

Chickpea Noodle Soup

Chickpeas are very high in fiber and are also rich in iron, folate, and protein.

INGREDIENTS:

- 2 cups chickpeas (also known as ceci or garbanzo beans)
- 4 cups water or vegetable stock
- 6 ounces fresh or dried pappardelle
- ⅓ cup extra virgin olive oil
- dash of sea salt

DIRECTIONS:

Soak beans overnight, and rinse before using (alternatively, you could use canned beans). In a large saucepan, bring the stock and beans to a simmer and cook until the beans are done. Taste and season with salt — you will need more or less depending on your stock. For a thicker broth, puree ½ cup of cooked beans in the blender and return to the pot. While the beans are cooking, boil the pappardelle in well-salted water. Drain and set aside ⅓ of the cooked noodles, and keep two cups of the pasta water in case you need additional liquid for the soup. Add the boiled noodles into the bean pot, and, depending on your preference, add the reserved pasta water if you want a bit more broth.

Meanwhile, in a large, heavy skillet, heat the olive oil. Fry the reserved noodles until crispy, but don't let the oil get too hot — it should be nicely fragrant. Drain the fried noodles on a paper towel and stir in two to three tablespoons of the olive oil into the soup. Serve with a generous sprinkling of the fried noodles mixed in at the last minute, and finish with a drizzle of your favorite olive oil.

San Francisco Cioppino

A great soup for a group! This fish stew cooked with tomatoes, wine and seafood has been associated with the San Francisco Bay Area since the 1930s when the Italian immigrants of San Francisco sold bowls of it full of crabmeat out of carts in the city streets. Don't skimp on the seafood; it is a healthy way to get your vitamins and nutrients. For example, mussels are a great source of vitamin B12, zinc and folate; whereas shrimp are high in calcium and protein.

INGREDIENTS:

- ¾ cup butter
- 2 onions, chopped
- 2 cloves garlic, minced
- 1 bunch fresh parsley, chopped
- 2 cans stewed tomatoes (14.5 ounce)
- 4 cups chicken broth
- 2 bay leaves
- 1 tbsp. dried basil
- ½ tsp. dried thyme
- ½ tsp. dried oregano
- 1 cup water
- 1½ cups white wine
- 1½ pounds large shrimp, peeled and deveined
- ½ pounds bay scallops
- 18 small clams
- 18 mussels, cleaned and de-bearded
- 1½ cups crabmeat
- 1½ pounds cod fillets, cubed (optional)

(Continued on next page.)

DIRECTIONS:

Over medium-low heat, melt butter in a large stockpot. Add onions, garlic and parsley, cooking slowly and stirring occasionally until onions are soft. Add tomatoes to the pot, breaking them into chunks, followed by the chicken broth, bay leaves, basil, thyme, oregano, water, and wine. Mix well; cover and simmer for 30 minutes. Stir in the shrimp, scallops, clams, mussels, and crabmeat. Stir in fish, if desired. Bring to boil, then reduce the heat to a simmer. Cover and simmer five to seven minutes, until the clams and mussels open. Ladle soup into bowls and serve with warm bread.

Creamed Broccoli and Mushroom Soup

This is a delicious and easy recipe that's great on cold winter days. Use fresh ingredients when possible, but you can use frozen or canned items if you wish. While mushrooms add flavor to this soup, they also add significant fiber and many of the B vitamins.

INGREDIENTS:

- 3 cups water
- 2 cups broccoli, chopped
- 1 cup mushrooms, sliced
- 2 tbsp. butter
- 1 cup nonfat dry milk powder
- 1 can condensed cheddar cheese soup (10.75 ounce)
- 2 dashes hot sauce
- ⅛ tsp. ground black pepper
- 1 dash garlic powder

DIRECTIONS:

In a large pot, add the water, broccoli, mushrooms, and butter and bring to a boil. Reduce heat to low, simmering five minutes, or until broccoli is tender. Mix in milk powder, condensed soup, hot sauce, pepper, and garlic powder. Continue cooking, stirring frequently, until heated thoroughly.

Ham and Potato Soup

INGREDIENTS:

- 3½ cups potatoes, peeled and diced
- ⅓ cup celery, diced
- ⅓ cup onion, finely chopped
- ¾ cup cooked ham, chopped
- 3¼ cups water
- 2 tbsp. chicken bouillon granules
- ½ tsp. salt
- 1 tbsp. ground black pepper
- 5 tbsp. butter
- 5 tbsp. all-purpose flour
- 2 cups milk

DIRECTIONS:

Combine the potatoes, celery, onion, ham, and water in a stockpot. Bring to a boil, then reduce the heat to medium and cook until potatoes are tender, about 10-15 minutes. Stir in the chicken bouillon, salt and pepper. In a separate saucepan, melt butter over low heat. Whisk in flour with a fork, and cook, stirring continually until thick, about 1 minute. Slowly stir in milk, a little at a time, as not to allow lumps to form. Continue stirring until thick, four to five minutes. Add the thickened milk mixture to the stockpot, and cook soup until heated thoroughly.

Harira (Moroccan Lamb Soup)

Harira is a traditional Moroccan soup usually served during Ramadan, the Muslim holy month, or on special occasions such as weddings. The combination of herbs and spices create a very interesting, flavorful aroma. So it's special, it's rare, it's exotic, but the main idea behind including this soup is to get you to eat lamb. Lamb is a delicious, lean meat high in iron, zinc and protein. It also contains high levels of vitamins B12 and B3, which aid in tissue development and in keeping the nervous system healthy!

INGREDIENTS:

- 1 lb. lamb meat, cubed
- 1 tsp. ground turmeric
- 1½ tsp. ground black pepper
- 1 tsp. ground cinnamon
- ¼ tsp. ground ginger
- ¼ tsp. ground cayenne pepper
- 2 tbsp. margarine
- ¾ cup chopped celery
- 1 onion, chopped
- 1 red onion, chopped
- ½ cup chopped fresh cilantro
- 1 can diced tomatoes (29 ounce)
- 7 cups water
- ¾ cup green lentils
- 1 can chickpeas, drained (15 ounce)
- 4 ounces vermicelli pasta
- 2 eggs, beaten
- 1 tbsp. fresh lemon juice

(Continued on next page.)

DIRECTIONS:

Place the lamb, spices, margarine in a large soup pot over a low heat, until the meat is slightly browned. Add the celery, onion, and cilantro and cook, stirring frequently, for five minutes. Pour tomatoes (reserve the juice) into the mixture and let simmer for 15 minutes. Add the reserved tomato juice, water and lentils to the pot. Bring the mixture to a boil, then reduce heat, simmering the soup, covered, for two hours. About 10 minutes before serving, turn the heat to medium-high, and add the chickpeas and noodles to the soup. Cook for about 10 minutes, or until noodles are al dente. Finally, stir in lemon juice and eggs, letting the eggs cook for a few minutes.

Indian Mulligatawny Soup

This delicious Anglo-Indian soup is a product of the notorious 18th century British Raj in India. The name "Mulligatawny" is an English version of the Indian phrase for "pepper water." Originally it was a rich, curried soup made with peppers, chicken stock, coconut milk, apples, almonds, chunks of chicken, and various vegetables. Our version is much healthier, opting for less cream, no coconut milk, and organic veggies. We also suggest spot-sautéing the vegetables to prevent losing the vitamins found therein. Serve it with Basmati rice or with a piece of Naan bread! You'll understand why the British stole the recipe and made it theirs.

INGREDIENTS:

- ½ cup onion, chopped
- 2 stalks celery, chopped
- 1 carrot, diced
- ¼ cup butter
- 1½ tbsp. all-purpose flour
- 1½ tsp. curry powder
- 4 cups organic chicken broth
- ½ apple, cored and chopped
- ¼ cup white rice
- 1 skinless, boneless chicken breast, cubed
- salt, to taste
- ground black pepper, to taste
- 1 pinch dried thyme
- ½ cup heavy cream, heated

DIRECTIONS:

Sauté onions, celery, carrot, and butter in a large stockpot. Add flour and curry, and cook five more minutes. Add chicken stock, mix well and bring to a boil. Simmer about 30 minutes. Then, add the apple, rice, chicken, salt, pepper, and thyme, simmering 15-20 minutes, or until rice is done. Add hot cream just before serving.

Italian Sausage Soup

What we love about this soup is that it tastes like it's been simmered all day, but it takes minutes to prepare in the microwave! Use only fresh herbs and use them sparingly.

INGREDIENTS:

- 1 lb. Italian sausage
- 1 clove garlic, minced
- 3½ cups beef broth
- 1 can Italian-style stewed tomatoes (14.5 ounce)
- 1 cup carrots, sliced
- 1 can Great Northern beans, undrained (14.5 ounce)
- 2 small zucchini, cubed
- 2 cups spinach, packed, rinsed and torn
- ¼ tsp. ground black pepper
- ¼ tsp. salt
- ¼ cup fresh basil
- grated Parmesan cheese, as a garnish

DIRECTIONS:

Cut sausage into ½-inch rounds. Brown on cooktop. Place sausage in a three- to four-quart microwave-safe casserole dish, along with garlic. Microwave on high power for two to three minutes, or until garlic is slightly softened. Add wine, tomatoes and juice, beef broth and fresh basil. Microwave on medium power (50%) for 15 minutes. Cool for a minute in refrigerator. Skim off the fat layer. Add pepper, zucchini, and beans. Microwave on high power again, covered, for 12 to 15 minutes or until beans are tender. Serve topped with the grated Parmesan cheese. For a heartier version of this soup, add tortellini. This soup recipe makes enough for six hearty servings. Enjoy!

Lentil Soup

For years lentils have been known to stabilize blood sugar, prevent heart disease, and provide an enormous source of iron. But lentils are also a natural alternative treatment for anxiety and depression thanks to the B vitamins they contain. Lentils are added to sautéed onions, carrots and celery. Lots of crushed tomatoes and water are added, and the magic begins. An hour later the soup is thick and wonderful and ready for a bit of shredded fresh spinach and a splash of vinegar. It's a tasty way to keep the blues away!

INGREDIENTS:

- 1 onion, chopped
- ¼ cup olive oil
- 2 carrots, diced
- 2 stalks celery, chopped
- 2 cloves garlic, minced
- 1 tsp. dried oregano
- 1 bay leaf
- 1 tsp. dried basil
- 1 can crushed tomatoes (14.5 ounce)
- 2 cups dry lentils
- 8 cups water
- ½ cup spinach, rinsed and thinly sliced
- 2 tbsp. vinegar
- salt, to taste
- ground black pepper, to taste

DIRECTIONS:

In a large soup pot, heat oil over medium heat. Add onions, carrots and celery; cook and stir until onion is tender. Stir in garlic, bay leaf, oregano, and basil; cook for two minutes. Add lentils, water, and tomatoes, and bring to a boil. Reduce heat and simmer for at least 1 hour. When ready to serve, stir in spinach, cooking until it wilts. Stir in vinegar, and season to taste with salt and pepper. More vinegar can be added, if desired.

Quick and Easy Chicken Noodle Soup

Chicken soup has been used as a cure for the common cold as far back as ancient Egypt. Modern research shows that there is some scientific basis for the belief in the curative powers of chicken soup. They found that the particular blend of nutrients and vitamins in traditional chicken soup slow the activity of certain white blood cells. This may have an anti-inflammatory effect that could hypothetically lead to temporary ease from symptoms of illness. Chicken soup is a good food for ventilating the nasal passages and clearing the sinuses, serving as a natural decongestant. Therefore, it does indeed relieve cold and flu symptoms.

INGREDIENTS:

- 1 tbsp. butter
- ½ cup onion, chopped
- ½ cup celery, chopped
- 7 cups organic chicken broth
- 1½ cups vegetable broth
- ½ lb. cooked chicken breast, chopped
- 1½ cups whole wheat elbow macaroni
- 1 cup carrots, sliced
- ½ tsp. dried basil
- ½ tsp. dried oregano
- salt and pepper, to taste

DIRECTIONS:

In a large pot over medium heat, melt butter. Cook onion and celery in the butter until just tender, about five minutes. Add all remaining ingredients to the pot, bringing it to a boil before reducing the heat. Simmer 20 minutes before serving. Delicious!

Split Pea Soup

Unlike other versions, this soup is absolutely vegetarian and exceptionally healthy! This green legume is loaded with folate, vitamins A, B1, B6, C, and a super-sized serving of osteoporosis-fighting K. Plus, they're a good source of vegetable protein. One cup of boiled green peas has 46% of your RDA of vitamin K1, known for maintaining bone health and — more important after surgery — helping blood to clot to prevent bleeding. So, all we are saying is, "Give peas a chance!"

INGREDIENTS:

- 2 tbsp. vegetable oil
- 4 cloves garlic, crushed
- 6 cups water
- ⅓ cup olive oil
- 3 cups dry green split peas
- 3 sprigs fresh parsley
- 1 dried red chili pepper
- 2 tsp. paprika
- 1 tsp. cumin
- 1 pinch salt
- 1 pinch black pepper

DIRECTIONS:

In a large pot over low heat, saute garlic in the vegetable oil until lightly browned. Pour in water and olive oil; stir in split peas, parsley, chili pepper, paprika, cumin, salt, and pepper. Bring to a boil, then reduce to low heat and simmer for about an hour, stirring occasionally so the peas do not stick to the bottom of the pot. When the peas are tender, mash them with a wooden spoon until smooth, while still in the pot. Stir in additional water to reach desired consistency.

Taco Soup

INGREDIENTS:

- 2 lbs. lean ground beef
- 1 onion, chopped
- ½ cup diced green chili
- 1 tsp. salt
- 1 tsp. ground black pepper
- 1 can pinto beans, drained (15 ounce)
- 1 can lima beans, drained (15 ounce)
- 1 pkg. taco seasoning mix (1.25 ounce)
- 1½ cups water
- 1 pkg. ranch dressing mix (1 ounce)
- 1 can white hominy, drained (15 ounce)
- 1 can stewed tomatoes (14.5 ounce)
- 1 can kidney beans, drained and rinsed (15 ounce)

DIRECTIONS:

In a large Dutch oven, brown the beef and chopped onion over medium heat. Drain off any fat. Add all the remaining ingredients to the beef and onion and bring to a boil. Reduce heat and simmer for 30 minutes. Top with shredded cheese and serve with chips.

Texas Corn Chowder

Jalapeno is very high in vitamins A, C and K, and it's a good source of vitamin E.

INGREDIENTS:

- ¼ cup onion, chopped
- 1 tbsp. butter
- 1 tbsp. all-purpose flour
- 1 cup potato, peeled and diced
- 1 cup water
- 1 cube chicken bouillon
- 1 cup fresh or frozen corn
- 1 tsp. jalapeno or other hot, green peppers, finely chopped
- 2 cups milk
- ¼ tsp. garlic salt
- ⅛ tsp. pepper
- 1 dash paprika

DIRECTIONS:

In a medium saucepan, saute onion in butter until tender. Stir in flour and cook for one minute. Add the potato, water, and bouillon and bring to a boil. Reduce heat; cover and simmer for 10 minutes or until potatoes are tender. Add corn, jalapeno, milk, and seasonings. Cover and simmer 15 minutes.

Tortilla and Bean Soup

Hominy and beans add a nice, smooth texture to this spice-filled soup. The tomatoes provide a good source of vitamin C and lycopene, a powerful antioxidant.

INGREDIENTS:

- 6 cups water
- 4 skinless, boneless chicken breasts
- 1 onion, chopped
- 1 can kidney beans (15 ounce)
- 1 can ranch-style beans (15 ounce)
- 1 can pinto beans (15 ounce)
- 1 can black beans, rinsed and drained (15 ounce)
- 1 can white hominy (15 ounce)
- 2 cans diced tomatoes with green chili peppers (10 ounces each)
- 1 pkg. taco seasoning mix (1.25 ounce)
- 1 pkg. ranch dressing mix (1 ounce)

DIRECTIONS:

Combine the chicken and water in a large pot over high heat. Cook for 30 minutes or up to one hour, or until chicken is fully cooked. Remove the meat from the pot and cut into bite-size pieces. Once chopped, return chicken to the pot and add the remainder of the ingredients. Mix well, reduce heat to low, and simmer for 30 minutes or until heated throughout.

Vegetable Soup

INGREDIENTS:

- 2 tsp. butter
- ½ cup onion, chopped
- 2 medium carrots, peeled, sliced and halved
- 2 medium potatoes, peeled and chopped
- 1 cup green beans, cut into 1-inch pieces
- 4 cups chicken broth
- 1 tbsp. chopped fresh parsley
- 1 tsp. dried tarragon leaves
- ¼ tsp. ground black pepper

DIRECTIONS:

Add butter to a large saucepan and stir in onion and carrots, cooking on medium-high heat for five minutes or until tender. Add potatoes, green beans, broth and spices; mix well. Cook 10 minutes or until potatoes are tender, stirring frequently. You can serve this chunky, as is, or puree in a blender to serve it cold.

LUNCH AND DINNER

Chicken Pesto Pasta

Eating this delicious dish can also prevent infection. Basil, the main ingredient of pesto, is actually a natural, gentle sedative that helps to relieve high blood pressure and the symptoms of peptic ulcers. The unique array of volatile oils found in basil — which contain estragole, linalool, cineole, eugenol, sabinene, myrcene, and limonene — provide protection against unwanted bacterial growth. Some bacteria that basil works best against are strains of bacteria from the genera Staphylococcus, Enterococcus and Pseudomonas, all of which are not only widespread but have now developed a high level of resistance to antibiotics.

INGREDIENTS:

- 2 tbsp. vegetable oil
- 2 boneless, skinless chicken breasts, chopped
- 1 tbsp. salt
- 8 oz. fettuccini
- 2½ cups basil
- 5 cloves garlic
- ½ cup pine nuts
- ⅔ cup olive oil
- ½ cup Parmesan cheese, grated

DIRECTIONS:

In a frying pan, heat the vegetable oil, and add the chopped chicken. Saute the meat and fully cook the chicken before setting it aside. To make the sauce, combine the basil, garlic and pine nuts in a food processor (or blender) until it reaches a paste-like texture. Slowly pour in the olive oil while still blending together. Then, stir in the cheese. Taste and season with salt and pepper, as needed. At the same time, boil a large pot of salted water. When it reaches a rolling boil, add the fettuccini and cook until al dente. Toss the cooked pasta with the pesto sauce, topping the dish with the cooked chicken pieces.

Chickpea Hot Pot

As a source of protein for the repair of muscles and as a source of fiber, it's hard to beat the chickpea. What makes it even more interesting is its versatility. Chickpeas can function as main courses or appetizers and in many forms and consistencies. Kale, full of antioxidants, comes from the cabbage family and has anti-inflammatory qualities. It is also high in vitamins A, K and C. Here is one of our favorite recipes that incorporates both.

INGREDIENTS:

- 1 large yellow onion, chopped
- a splash of olive oil
- a couple pinches of salt
- ⅔ cup uncooked bulgur
- 1 can of chickpeas, drained and rinsed (14 ounce)
- 4½ cups vegetable stock
- ½ cup orange juice
- 1½ cup cauliflower, trimmed into small trees
- 2 cups kale, de-stemmed and cut into thin ribbons
- olive oil, for garnish
- red onion, chopped, for garnish

DIRECTIONS:

In a large pot over medium heat, saute the onion in olive oil, seasoned with salt, until softened. Stir in the bulgur, chickpeas and stock, bringing the ingredients to a simmer. Cook for a few minutes — it should start to thicken. Taste to see if the bulgur is cooked through. If so, continue; if not, continue simmering until cooked. Add the orange juice, cauliflower and kale, simmering another few minutes, until the cauliflower is just tender. If the stew is on the thick side, thin with additional water or stock. Once served, garnish with a drizzle of olive oil and chopped red onions.

Fish in Foil

What's fishy about wanting to enjoy good health? Rainbow trout is an excellent choice because it is lower in fat and calories than some foods from the meat group and also is a good source of many important nutrients. A 3-ounce serving of cooked rainbow trout contains 22 grams of protein and only 130 calories, 4 grams of fat, and very little sodium.

INGREDIENTS:

- 2 rainbow trout fillets
- 1 tbsp. olive oil
- 2 tsp. garlic salt
- 1 tsp. ground black pepper
- 1 fresh jalapeno pepper, sliced
- 1 lemon, sliced

DIRECTIONS:

Preheat oven to 400°. Rinse fish and pat dry. Rub fillets with olive oil and season with garlic salt and black pepper. Place each fillet on a large sheet of aluminum foil. Top with jalapeno slices and squeeze the juice from the ends of the lemon over the fish. Arrange lemon slices on top of fillets. Carefully seal all edges of the foil to form enclosed packets and place the packets on a baking sheet. Bake for 15-20 minutes, depending on the size of fish. Fish is done when it flakes easily with a fork.

Frittata

This crustless version of the quiche is a sophisticated treat. Plus, eggs are a great source of protein and easy to chew after dental surgery.

INGREDIENTS:

- 1 tbsp. olive oil
- ½ cup onion, diced
- 1 10-ounce package frozen spinach, thawed and squeezed dry
- ½ cup cooked potato, diced
- ½ cup herbed goat cheese, crumbled
- 6 eggs, slightly beaten
- 1 tsp. salt
- 1 tsp. pepper

DIRECTIONS:

In a small frying pan over low heat, sauté the onion in olive oil until soft. Then, evenly distribute the sliced potato and goat cheese around the pan. Add eggs, seasoned with salt and pepper, to the frying pan, covering the cheese and vegetables. Cook on low-medium heat until most of the egg has set. Then flip the egg mixture over to finish cooking the other side. Best served with toast.

Lamb and Winter Vegetable Stew

We like cooking but we can be a little bit impatient. Parsnips and sweet potatoes add depth to this stew; parsnips also add potassium and fiber, while the sweet potato is abundant in vitamin A. This is a great recipe for good health.

INGREDIENTS:
- 2 tbsp. vegetable oil
- 1 lb. lamb stew meat, cubed
- 2 cups beef broth
- 1 cup dry red wine
- 2 cloves garlic, minced
- 1 tbsp. fresh thyme, chopped
- ¼ tsp. salt
- ¼ tsp. black pepper
- 1 bay leaf
- 2 cups butternut squash, peeled, seeded and sliced
- 1 cup parsnips, peeled and sliced
- 1 cup sweet potatoes, peeled and chopped
- 1 cup celery, sliced
- 1 medium onion, thinly sliced
- ½ cup sour cream
- 3 tbsp. all-purpose flour

DIRECTIONS:

Heat the oil in a large saucepan, and brown the lamb on all sides. Drain fat, and stir in the beef broth and wine. Add the spices and bring the mixture to a boil. Reduce heat, cover, and simmer 20 minutes. Mix in the squash, parsnips, sweet potatoes, celery, and onion. Again, bring to a boil, then reduce heat and simmer for 30 minutes, or until the vegetables are tender. In a small bowl, blend the sour cream and flour together. Slowly stir in ½ cup of the hot stew mixture into the sour cream blend. Then stir the sour cream mix into the stew. Remove the bay leaf, and continue to cook until thickened, stirring often.

Mediterranean Fish Stew

Not to be confused with its counterpart — the classic "marin" bouillabaisse from Marseille that is famous for its aromatic combination of fennel seeds, saffron and orange zest — this stew is much more humble. While French gourmets sing the praises of the former, this is the one fishermen actually eat all the time. This simple, hearty fish stew is all you need for omega-3s, to help build muscle and cardiovascular health.

INGREDIENTS:

- 4 cloves garlic, minced
- 2 onions, chopped
- 1 tbsp. olive oil
- 1 can crushed tomatoes (28 ounce)
- 6 cups water
- ½ cup fresh parsley, chopped
- ½ cup fresh cilantro, chopped
- 2 tbsp. Worcestershire sauce
- 1 tsp. ground cinnamon
- 1 tsp. paprika
- 1½ lbs. cod fillets, cubed
- 3 ounces dry pasta
- salt, to taste
- 1 tbsp. ground black pepper

DIRECTIONS:

In a large pot over medium heat, saute the garlic and onions in the olive oil for five minutes, stirring constantly. Add the tomatoes (including their liquid), water, parsley, and cilantro. Bring to a boil, then reduce heat to low and simmer for 15 minutes. Stir in the Worcestershire sauce, cinnamon, paprika and fish, simmering over medium heat for 10 minutes. Add the pasta and simmer for an additional 8 minutes, or until pasta is tender. Season with salt to taste and ground black pepper.

Okra Stew with Shrimp

What do okra and yogurt have in common? They both facilitate the propagation of good bacteria, referred to as probiotics, in the small intestine. This Southern meal acts as an excellent laxative for irritable bowels and soothes the gastrointestinal track. Okra is a good source of fiber and also provides vitamins C, A, and calcium.

INGREDIENTS:

- 1 lb. medium shrimp, peeled and deveined
- 2 tsp. lime juice
- 4 tbsp. butter
- 2 green bell peppers, seeded
- 6 tbsp. minced shallots
- 1 cup corn kernels, frozen
- 1 cup okra, chopped
- 3 tomatoes, blanched, peeled and chopped
- 1 tbsp. tomato paste
- ¼ tsp. dried thyme
- 1 bay leaf
- 1 green chili pepper
- salt and pepper, to taste

DIRECTIONS:

Place shrimp in mixing bowl and toss with lime juice, coating evenly. Heat butter in a stock pot and saute the green peppers and shallots for three minutes. Mix in corn, okra, tomatoes, tomato paste, thyme, bay leaf, and chilli pepper. Season with salt and pepper, and simmer for 10 minutes. Add the shrimp, and return to a boil, then simmer for another five minutes until shrimp is cooked. Remove the bay leaf and chili pepper before serving.

Orzo Shrimp Stew

Orzo is often thought of as "Italian rice," yet it is simply small rice-shaped pasta full of carbs and protein.

INGREDIENTS:

- 2½ cups chicken broth
- 5 cups broccoli florets
- 1 can diced tomatoes, undrained (14.5 ounce)
- 1 cup uncooked orzo
- 1 lb. uncooked medium shrimp, peeled and deveined
- ¾ tsp. salt
- ¼ tsp. pepper
- 2 tsp. dried basil
- 2 tbsp. butter

DIRECTIONS:

In a large nonstick saucepan, bring the broth to a boil. Add the broccoli, tomatoes, and orzo, and reduce heat to a simmer. Cook uncovered for five minutes, stirring occasionally. Add the shrimp, salt and pepper and cover, cooking for four to five minutes or until shrimp turns pink and orzo is tender. Stir in basil and butter to finish.

Quiche

Real men do eat quiche, despite what clichés intimate. Real men who worked the farmlands in Germany in a medieval town known as Lothringen, where this hearty staple was invented, ate this "cake" after toiling in the fields all day. Real men in the British army ate this "pie" filled with meats because it was cheap and filling. It was only after quiche landed in America via France that it somehow became known as a "light and fluffy" dish. All we can tell you is that must have been some good marketing because quiche is actually very hearty and heavy. This classic recipe is also rich in calcium, helping your digestive system and strengthening your bones.

INGREDIENTS:

- 1 cup chopped bacon
- ½ pkg. frozen chopped spinach, thawed (use 5 ounces)
- 2 tbsp. olive oil
- ½ onion, finely diced
- ½ cup sour cream
- ½ tsp. salt
- 1 tsp. pepper
- 1 unbaked 9-inch pie crust
- 1 cup cheddar cheese, shredded
- ¼ cup Parmesan cheese, grated
- 4 eggs
- ¾ cup half and half
- 1 tsp. dried parsley
- salt and pepper to taste

(Continued on next page.)

DIRECTIONS:

Preheat oven to 375°. Cook bacon in a large, deep skillet over medium-high heat. Drain, crumble, and set aside. Cook spinach according to the package instructions. Allow to cool, and squeeze dry. Heat olive oil in a skillet over medium heat, cooking the onion until soft and translucent. Then, add in the crumbled bacon to the onion mixture and remove from heat. In a large bowl, combine spinach, sour cream, salt, and pepper. Spread the spinach mixture into the pie crust. Next, layer the bacon, followed by the cheddar and parmesan cheese. Whisk together the eggs, cream, parsley, salt, and pepper, and pour over the pie shell. Place the pie on a baking sheet, and bake on the middle shelf for 40 minutes. The top will be puffed and golden brown. Remove from oven, and let stand for 10 minutes.

Rajasthani Buttermilk Curry

We personally recommend this dish because of its healing properties. Turmeric, which gives curry its yellow color, contains curcuminoid, a property known to help prevent Alzheimer's and arthritis, reducing any inflammation of joints and muscles. But recently, studies have shown it also may prevent asthma, multiple sclerosis, and osteoporosis. Try using a yogurt that has probiotic cultures, which provide "good" bacteria to aid digestion. This authentic dish will make you feel like you traveled all the way to India to taste it.

INGREDIENTS:

- 1 tbsp. vegetable oil
- 1½ tsp. black mustard seeds
- ½ tsp. cumin seeds
- ½ tsp. turmeric
- 2 medium scallions, trimmed and sliced
- 1 green cayenne pepper, minced
- 1 cup plain yogurt OR 1¼ cups buttermilk
- ¼ cup water, if using yogurt
- ½ tsp. salt
- ⅔ tbsp. chopped cilantro

DIRECTIONS:

Heat oil in a wok or heavy pot over high heat. When hot, toss in mustard seeds. Then, once most have "popped," add cumin, turmeric and stir. Lower the heat to medium and add the scallions and peppers, stir-frying until softened, about three minutes. If using yogurt, stir in the water. Reduce the heat to low, and pour in the yogurt or butter milk. Stir until warmed throughout, but do not allow the mixture to boil. Stir in the salt and transfer to a serving bowl. Garnish with chopped cilantro.

DESSERTS
Apple Rhubarb Crumble

Rhubarb was brought to America from Europe in the late 1700s. Today there are more than 60 varieties of this interesting vegetable available. Folk remedies often used rhubarb to aid with indigestion and constipation. Today we also know rhubarb can regulate fat absorption. Got your attention now?

INGREDIENTS:

Filling:

- 2 cups apples, peeled, cored, sliced
- 2 cups rhubarb, chopped
- ¼ cup sugar
- ½ cup pecan pieces
- 1 tsp. cinnamon

Crumble:

- ¼ cup brown sugar
- ¼ cup flour
- dash of salt
- ¼ cup butter
- ¼ cup rolled oats

DIRECTIONS:

Preheat oven to 400°. In an oven-proof deep dish, mix together the fruit, sugar, pecans and cinnamon. In another bowl, combine the brown sugar, flour and salt. Cut in the butter with a fork until it looks crumbly. Add the rolled oats and sprinkle over the fruit mixture. Bake 30-40 minutes until golden brown on top.

Bread and Butter Pudding

This is essentially a baked form of French toast. Best when made with brioche and served warm with custard and cream. Perfect for tender gums.

INGREDIENTS:

- 4 cups white bread, diced
- ½ cup raisins
- ½ cup dried cranberries
- 2 eggs, slightly beaten
- 1¾ cups milk
- 2 tsp. vanilla
- 1 tsp. cinnamon
- ¾ cup sugar

DIRECTIONS:

Preheat oven to 350°. Fill a 9x9-inch pan with the bread pieces; scatter the bread with raisins and cranberries. In a mixing bowl, combine eggs, milk, vanilla, cinnamon, and sugar. Pour wet ingredients over the bread and let sit for five to 10 minutes, so the bread can absorb some of the liquid. Bake for 40-50 minutes, or until firm and colored on top. Let sit 10 more minutes before serving.

Strawberry Parfait

INGREDIENTS:

- 1 cup vanilla yogurt
- 1 cup granola
- 1 cup strawberries
- ½ cup whipped cream
- ¼ cup slivered almonds
- 2 sprigs of mint leaves

DIRECTIONS:

Using either parfait glasses or simply tall drink glasses, layer ¼ cup of yogurt, ¼ cup of granola and ¼ cup of strawberries; then repeat these layers again. Top with a dollop of whipped cream, slivered almonds and mint sprig. Complete the entire process again in a second glass. For added decadence, try drizzling chocolate sauce on top.

Very Berry Pie

Eat, drink and be berry! This pie will have any precancerous cells running for cover. Raspberries contain significant amounts of polyphenol antioxidants such as anthocyanin pigments. Buy the frozen organic berries: they work just as well as fresh. Raspberries are also a rich source of vitamin C, about 50% of our daily-recommended value. Drench in delicious vanilla ice cream or custard. Enjoy!

INGREDIENTS:

- 2 unbaked 9-inch pie crusts
- 2 cups raspberries, fresh or frozen
- 1 cup strawberries, sliced, fresh or frozen
- 1 cup blueberries, fresh or frozen
- 1 tsp. lemon juice
- ¾ cup sugar
- ¼ cup flour
- 1 tbsp. butter

DIRECTIONS:

Preheat the oven to 400°. Mix together the berries and lemon juice in a large bowl. In another bowl, stir the sugar and flour together. Combine the dry ingredients with the fruit mixture, coating the berries evenly. Place berries in one of the pie shells and dot with small pieces of butter. Invert the second pie shell on top of the filled shell and pinch around the edges to seal. Cut several slits on the top of the pie, allowing steam to escape. Bake at 400° for 15 minutes, then reduce heat and bake at 375° for 45 minutes, until golden on top. Let rest 15 minutes before serving.

CHAPTER 4
Days 6–14

n addition to cooking many of the fine dishes from our previous menus, your mouth will now be ready to enjoy the nourishing and comforting meals below.

MAIN COURSES

Almond-Crusted Halibut Crystal Symphony *

Broiled Tilapia Parmesan *

Chicken Fettuccini Alfredo *

Fish in Ginger-Tamarind Sauce *

Grilled Salmon Kyoto *

Lasagna *

Orange Roughy *

Salmon Patties *

Sesame Seared Tuna *

All of the fish in these dishes are a good source of protein and, of course, contain omega-3 fatty acids, which are known to benefit your cardiovascular system and your nervous system. Fatty fish, in particular, is recommended to be eaten at least twice a week.

Almond-Crusted Halibut Crystal Symphony

INGREDIENTS:

Sauce:

- ⅓ cup dry white wine
- 2 tbsp. cider vinegar
- 2 tbsp. shallots, minced
- 1 sprig fresh thyme
- 1 bay leaf
- ⅓ cup heavy cream
- ½ cup unsalted butter, chilled, chopped
- 3 tbsp. fresh chives, chopped
- 2 tsp. lemon juice
- salt and pepper, to taste

Fish:

- 6 6-ounce halibut fillets, between ¾ and 1 inch thick
- 2 tbsp. vegetable oil
- 1 tbsp. unsalted butter
- ¼ cup breadcrumbs
- ⅔ cup blanched almonds, minced
- 1 tbsp. unsalted butter, melted
- 1 egg, lightly beaten

DIRECTIONS:

Begin by making a beurre blanc sauce: In a small saucepan over
medium heat, combine wine, vinegar, shallots, thyme, and bay leaf.
Boil until almost all of the liquid has evaporated; then add the cream,
boiling until it is reduced by half. Turn the heat down low and whisk
in butter, one piece at a time. Don't allow sauce to simmer, or it may
separate. Next, strain the sauce through a fine sieve into a heatproof
bowl. Stir in chives and lemon juice, adding salt and pepper to taste.
While cooking the fish, keep the sauce warm by setting the bowl in a
larger container of hot water.

(Continued on next page.)

Preheat oven to broiler setting. Pat fillets dry, and season with salt and pepper. Meanwhile, heat oil and butter in a large skillet, over medium heat. When the oil is hot, saute the halibut fillets for two to three minutes a side, until lightly browned and just cooked through. Then, transfer the fish to a baking sheet, and let cool for five minutes. In a small bowl, stir together bread crumbs, almonds and melted butter; brush the top of each fillet with the beaten egg, and top that with the almond mixture. Broil for two minutes, or until browned — watch closely! To serve, place fillets on individual plates and spoon beurre blanc sauce around the fish.

Broiled Tilapia Parmesan

INGREDIENTS:

- ½ cup Parmesan cheese
- ¼ cup butter, softened
- 3 tbsp. mayonnaise
- 2 tbsp. lemon juice
- ¼ tsp. dried basil
- ¼ tsp. black pepper
- ⅛ tsp. onion powder
- ⅛ tsp. celery salt
- 2 lbs. tilapia fillets

DIRECTIONS:

Preheat oven to broiler setting. Grease a broiling pan or line it with aluminum foil. In a small bowl, mix together cheese, butter, mayonnaise, and lemon juice. Then stir in basil, pepper, onion powder and celery salt, and set aside. Arrange fillets in a single layer on the prepared pan. Broil three minutes a side, a few inches from the heat. Remove the fish from the oven and cover the top side with the cheese mixture. Broil until the topping is brown and fish flakes easily with a fork, about two minutes. Be careful not to overcook the fish!

Chicken Fettuccini Alfredo

INGREDIENTS:

- 6 boneless, skinless chicken breasts, cubed
- 1 tbsp. Italian seasoning
- 6 tbsp. butter
- 4 cloves garlic, minced
- 1 lb. fettuccini
- 1 onion, diced
- 1 pkg. sliced mushrooms (8 ounce)
- ⅓ cup all-purpose flour
- 1 tbsp. salt
- ¾ tsp. white pepper
- 3 cups milk
- 1 cup half and half
- ¾ cup Parmesan cheese, grated
- 2 cups Monterey Jack cheese, shredded
- 3 plum tomatoes, diced
- ½ cup sour cream

DIRECTIONS:

In a large skillet over medium heat, combine chicken, Italian seasoning, and two tablespoons each of butter and garlic. Fully cook the chicken and remove from the skillet and set aside (chicken should no longer be pink inside). Next, bring a large pot of lightly salted water to a boil; add pasta and cook 10 minutes or until al dente and drain. Meanwhile, melt four tablespoons of butter in the skillet; saute onion, remaining garlic, and mushrooms, cooking until onions are transparent. Stir in flour, salt, and pepper, cooking for two minutes. Slowly add milk and cream, stirring until smooth and creamy. Then, gradually add both cheeses and stir until melted. Finally, add chicken, tomatoes and sour cream. Serve over cooked fettuccini.

Fish in Ginger-Tamarind Sauce

INGREDIENTS:

- 1 tbsp. vegetable oil
- 1 tsp. mustard seed
- 2 tbsp. fresh ginger, chopped
- 1 cup onions, chopped
- 2 cups water
- 1 tbsp. tamarind paste
- 2 tbsp. coriander, ground
- ½ tsp. chili powder
- salt, to taste
- ½ lb. cod fillets, cut into 1-inch cubes
- fresh curry leaves (optional)

DIRECTIONS:

Heat oil in a saucepan over medium-high heat. When hot, add mustard seeds and cook until they begin to crackle. Then add ginger and onion, cooking until softened, about five minutes. Pour in water and add the tamarind paste. Bring this to a boil before adding coriander, chili powder, and salt. Reduce heat to medium-low and cook for 15 minutes, stirring occasionally. Add fish to the pan and cook thoroughly. Garnish with fresh curry leaves.

Grilled Salmon Kyoto

INGREDIENTS:

- ⅓ cup soy sauce
- ¼ cup orange juice concentrate
- 2 tbsp. vegetable oil
- 2 tbsp. tomato sauce
- 1 tsp. lemon juice
- ½ tsp. prepared mustard
- 1 tbsp. green onion, minced
- 1 clove garlic, minced
- ½ tsp. fresh ginger, minced
- 4 salmon steaks, 1 inch thick
- 1 tbsp. olive oil

DIRECTIONS:

In a shallow glass baking dish, combine all ingredients except salmon and olive oil. Then, place salmon in marinade and turn to coat. Cover and refrigerate for 30 minutes to one hour. Once the fish is almost ready, preheat an outdoor grill to high heat. Remove salmon from marinade, reserving the liquid in a small saucepan. Bring the liquid to a boil, and cook for one to two minutes. Next, lightly oil the grill grate and brush or spray salmon with olive oil. Place fish on the grill and cook for 10 minutes or until fish flakes easily with a fork. Turn salmon once, and brush with boiled marinade halfway through cooking time. Delicious fish, Japanese-style!

Lasagna

INGREDIENTS:

- 1 lb. sweet Italian sausage
- ¾ lb. lean ground beef
- ½ cup onion, minced
- 2 cloves garlic, crushed
- 1 can crushed tomatoes (28 ounce)
- 2 cans tomato paste (6 ounce)
- 2 cans tomato sauce (6.5 ounce)
- ½ cup water
- 2 tbsp. sugar
- 1½ tsp. dried basil leaves
- ½ tsp. fennel seeds
- 1 tsp. Italian seasoning
- 1 tbsp. salt
- ¼ tsp. black pepper
- 4 tbsp. fresh parsley, chopped
- 12 lasagna noodles
- 16 ounces ricotta cheese
- 1 egg
- ½ tsp. salt
- ¾ lb. mozzarella cheese, sliced
- ¾ cup grated Parmesan cheese

(Continued on next page.)

DIRECTIONS:

In a Dutch oven, cook sausage, ground beef, onion, and garlic over medium heat until well browned. Stir in crushed tomatoes, tomato paste, tomato sauce, and water. Season with sugar, basil, fennel seeds, Italian seasoning, salt, pepper, and half the parsley. Simmer, covered, for about 1½ hours, stirring occasionally. Afterwards, bring a large pot of lightly salted water to a boil. Add lasagna noodles to the water and cook about 10 minutes. Drain noodles and rinse with cold water. Meanwhile, in a mixing bowl, combine ricotta cheese with egg, remaining parsley and ½ teaspoon salt. Preheat oven to 375°.

Now you're ready to begin assembling the lasagna. First, spread 1½ cups of meat sauce in the bottom of a 9x13-inch baking dish. Then, arrange six noodles lengthwise over meat sauce. Spread with half of the ricotta cheese mixture, and top that with ⅓ of the mozzarella. Next, spoon 1½ cups of meat sauce over mozzarella, and sprinkle with ¼ cup of Parmesan. Repeat layers, and top with remaining mozzarella and Parmesan cheese. Cover with foil and bake for 25 minutes. (To prevent sticking, either spray foil with cooking spray or make sure the foil does not touch the cheese.) After the first 25 minutes remove foil, and bake another 25 minutes uncovered. Cool for 15 minutes before serving.

Orange Roughy

The orange roughy is a large deep-sea fish typically found in the cold, deep waters of the western Pacific Ocean, eastern Atlantic and Indo-Pacific. This fish is notable for its lengthy lifespan — 150 years — and bright red scales that fade to a yellowish orange by the time it arrives on your plate. Ridiculously low in fat, the orange roughy is also an excellent source of selenium, vitamin B12 and niacin.

INGREDIENTS:

- 1 tsp. olive oil
- 3 green onions, chopped
- 1 cup dry white wine
- 1 can whole peeled tomatoes with liquid, chopped (14.5 ounce)
- 4 4-ounce orange roughy fillets
- 1 tbsp. fresh basil, chopped
- ¼ tsp. black pepper
- 1 pinch dried thyme, crushed
- 1 pinch dried rosemary, crushed
- ¼ cup black olives, sliced and drained
- ½ lb. feta cheese, crumbled

DIRECTIONS:

To prepare, heat olive oil in a medium skillet over medium heat. Add green onions, and cook until tender, about five to 10 minutes. Then, stir in white wine and tomatoes and bring to a boil. Place the fish fillets in the white wine mixture, seasoning with basil, pepper, thyme, and rosemary. Reduce heat and simmer the fish 15-20 minutes, until fish is easily flaked with a fork. Remove fish fillets from skillet and top with black olives and feta cheese.

Salmon Patties

To benefit from antioxidants and omega-3 fatty acids, salmon is an ideal source.

INGREDIENTS:

- ½ lb. salmon
- 1 red potato, peeled and chopped
- 1 shallot, minced
- 1 egg, beaten
- ¼ cup Italian seasoned breadcrumbs
- 1 tsp. Italian seasoning
- salt and pepper, to taste
- ½ cup cornflake crumbs
- 2 tbsp. olive oil

DIRECTIONS:

Preheat oven to 350° and lightly grease a small baking dish. Place the salmon in the prepared baking dish; cover and bake 20 minutes, or until easily flaked with a fork. While the fish is cooking, boil the potato in a small saucepan and cook until tender, 10-15 minutes. Once cooked, drain and mash the potato. Next, combine the salmon, potato, shallot, egg, and breadcrumbs in a bowl, and add the Italian seasoning, salt, and pepper. In a separate bowl nearby, place the cornflake crumbs. Then, using the salmon mixture, create 1-inch balls of salmon. Roll the balls in the cornflakes to coat, and press into patties. Heat the olive oil in a medium saucepan, and fry the patties over medium heat, three to five minutes a side, or until golden brown. Delicious!

Sesame Seared Tuna

INGREDIENTS:

- ¼ cup soy sauce
- 1 tbsp. mirin (Japanese sweet wine)
- 1 tbsp. honey
- 2 tbsp. sesame oil
- 1 tbsp. rice wine vinegar
- 4 6-ounce tuna steaks
- ½ cup sesame seeds
- wasabi paste
- 1 tbsp. olive oil

DIRECTIONS:

In a small bowl, stir together soy sauce, mirin, honey and sesame oil. Divide the liquid into two equal parts. Stir the rice vinegar into one part and set this aside as a dipping sauce. Coat the tuna steaks with the remaining soy sauce mixture. Next, spread the sesame seeds out on a plate and press the tuna into them to coat. Heat the olive oil until very hot in a cast iron skillet on high heat. Place steaks in the pan, and sear for about 30 seconds on each side. Serve with the dipping sauce and wasabi paste.

CHAPTER 5

Day 14 and Beyond

Health and Nutrition

Congratulations! You made it. With a fantastic foundation built within the past two-week period where your mouth has had ample time to heal by eating softer, gum-sensitive nutritional food, you have now reached the 14-day marker, where you can resume a normal diet.

After Day 14 you can eat whatever you wish, but be careful not to disturb any residual swelling that might be present in the surgical site. Add solid foods to your diet as soon as they are comfortable to chew.

But now that you have conscientiously integrated this healthier eating regime into your life,we believe you will want to continue.

Oral health is a critical part of your overall health. Don't wait until the next dental surgery to focus on taking good care of your teeth and your gums.

Fitness 101

Your overall health and wellbeing are key to a speedy recovery process from any type of surgery, including dental surgery.

Along with healthy eating, as guided by the menus within the preceding chapters of this book, you should be conscious of the value of nutrition in your diet and the level of fitness in your daily activities. This ideal combination of a balanced amount of vitamins and nutrients along with regular exercise is critical for post-operative recovery. Not to mention, by being aware of both these factors, you can aim to stay at an optimum health level in the weeks, months and years to come.

You don't need to enlist a fitness trainer and nutritionist. All you need to do is follow a suitable plan that includes exercises, proper nutrition, and embracing a healthier lifestyle plan.

In the days following surgery, it will be natural to feel tired and achy, so common sense says that you shouldn't overexert yourself. This especially means taking care not to exacerbate sensitive or delicate areas; in this case, around your head and mouth area.

It's not recommended that you attempt any vigorous physical exercise that involves head-turning, nodding, neck strain, or inverting your body. For example, strenuous yoga positions, sit-ups, push-ups, or running might be too stressful in these early days of recovery.

However, a moderate amount of fitness and exercise will be a productive way to build your body into a stronger, fitter, and healthier machine.

Exercise has multiple benefits in addition to controlling weight: it can reduce the risk of cardiac disease, lower blood pressure, improve mental function, improve blood glucose levels, reduce the risk of some cancers, and improve the immune system. When it becomes apparent it is safe to do so, try to get at least 30 minutes of physical activity each day.

Physical activity is defined as activities in addition to your normal daily routines such as going to work, shopping, or housekeeping.

Running might be too hard on your body at this time, but fast walking or even a short walk around the block will be worthwhile and rewarding. In fact, you will be amazed at how good it will make you feel!

Five Pillars of Fitness

Supporting your entire fitness plan, the five pillars of fitness are essential elements for healthier, stronger and longer living.

Strength, agility, flexibility, cardiovascular, and endurance exercises should be included as part of every well-rounded and balanced fitness regime. Of course, there are many different exercises that can benefit each pillar from this group; however, all of the exercises that are specially recommended within these five pillars are intended as safe for post-operative patients who are 14 days into their recovery, and onwards.

However, if in doubt, or you do not feel 100% ready for this type of movement, please do not attempt it.

Strength

Building and toning muscles is what strength training is all about. This can involve using weights and repetitions of movement — essentially, fewer reps can be performed with heavier weights to achieve results similar to more reps with lighter weights.

Ultimately, strength training is about completing the action not once or twice, but repeating it 6 to 12 times (called a "set"). This helps to develop strength and endurance.

Types of weight equipment can include barbells, dumbbells, and even using your own body weight by performing chin-ups and push-ups.

Push-Ups

Target Area: chest and arms (pectoral, triceps, biceps)

In a classic push-up, you lie flat, face down on the floor, with your stomach to the ground; bring your hands up to your shoulders and raise your toes, so the bottom of your toes touch the ground.

With your legs out straight behind you, push up, keeping your back straight and stomach tight. Then, lower yourself in this horizontal position until your elbows make a right angle and/or your chest almost reaches the floor.

VARIATION: If this is a challenge, try with your knees bent to begin with, gradually working up to a full-body push-up.

Are you improving? Once a month, do as many push-ups as possible to find out your maximum repetition level. This number should increase over time, with more practice and training.

Crunches

Target Area: Abdominal muscles

Lie on the floor, face up, with your back flat and knees bent, so the soles of your feet are flat on the floor.

Place your arms gently behind your head. Curl your neck and shoulders up off the floor and feel your abdominal muscles "crunch." Then, release and lower your shoulders back down. You should be using your abdominals, not your arms, to curl you up. There should be no pull on your neck.

VARIATION: Try raising your legs in the air, with bended knees; keep your legs in this position throughout the crunch. Alternatively, try lifting only one shoulder and twisting to target the oblique abdominal muscles; be sure to crunch both sides.

Are you improving? Once a month, do as many crunches as possible to find out your maximum repetition level. This number should increase over time, with more practice and training.

Squats

Target Area: lower body (quadriceps, hamstrings, calves and gluts)

The idea of a squat is basically bending your knees and rising again. To begin, start with your feet shoulder width apart; bend your knees and squat as low as possible.

During your bend, bring your arms out in front of you, parallel with the floor. Then straighten back up to a standing position again; and repeat.

VARIATION: For more of a challenge, try it on one leg. Support yourself on one leg and lift the other in front of you while bending. Be sure to repeat on the other leg.

Are you improving? Once a month, do as many squats as possible to find out your Maximum Repetition level. This number should increase over time, with more practice and training. Also, you may notice a difference in the level of squat that you can achieve; with time, you may be able to bend lower, into a deeper squat.

Lunges

Target Area: glutes, hamstrings

To try this lunge, stand with one foot in front of the next, 2-3 feet apart. The goal is to have both knees at a 90° angle when you're bending your knees, so you may need to bring your feet closer or further apart.

To begin, bend your knees: your front heel stays down on the floor, with the knee directly over the foot, while the back leg/knee is lowered towards the floor. Your upper body should remain straight throughout the movement. Then, push up through your front foot and return to the starting position, keeping your knees bent slightly in the top position. Try doing 2-3 sets of 10-15 repetitions.

VARIATION: As you increase your level of strength and comfort with this exercise, add extra weight. For instance, hold hand weights in each hand as you perform this exercise. If you don't have barbells, try a can of soup or bottle of water in each hand instead.

Are you improving? Once a month, do as many lunges as possible to find out your Maximum Repetition level. This number should increase over time, with more practice and training.

Leg Lift

Target Area: lower body (legs, hips, abs)

Lie on the floor, face up, on your back, placing your hands under your hips; your legs should be straight in front of you. Slowly lift one leg off the floor, about six inches high, and hold it in the air. Then, lower and repeat with the other leg.

Once this movement is comfortable, try raising both legs off the ground together. When they're in the air, spread your legs out wide and then bring them back together; then lower them to the ground.

VARIATION: Instead of spreading your legs apart, simply keep them hovering six inches off the ground and hold this position for 30-45 seconds before lowering.

Are you improving? Continue until your strength improves to desired level.

Lifestyle activities which also encourage strength:
weightlifting, swimming, rowing.

Agility

Agility is all about being able quickly to change the direction your body is headed. This requires a combination of balance, coordination, reflexes and speed — particularly useful when playing racket sports, for instance.

Shuttle Run

This exercise has you run in one direction, then another, and back again. Mark two parallel lines on the floor, about 10 feet apart (try using a piece of tape on the floor to mark the lines). Starting in the middle of the lines, run towards the left line and touch it; then run towards the opposite line, and touch it, before finally running back to the first line.

You can do this back-and-forth shuttle for a set amount of time, or you can time yourself for three or five re-directions, and try to beat your time.

VARIATION: Change the footwork. Try doing this drill running forwards and backwards between lines, doing a side-step, side to side between lines, or even running sideways, crossing your feet in front and behind with each step.

Are you improving? Either count how many re-directions you can do in a set period, i.e., 1 minute, or see how fast you can complete a series of re-directions, continually trying to beat your previous time.

Ski Hops

Draw two lines, 10 meters long and 1 meter apart. Looking up the length of both lines, and starting on the far side of one line, jump horizontally across to the outside of the other line (so you're jumping over both lines). Jump back and forth, from one side to the next as you move down the length of the lines. When you reach the end, turn around and repeat the exercise.

VARIATION: Face the lines so that you're looking horizontally across both of them. Starting on the far side and at one end, jump forward, across both lines, and then jump backwards trying to jump across both lines. Repeat all the way up the lines.

Are you improving? Depending on your agility, having the lines at 1 meter apart may be too challenging; if so, consider bring the lines in slightly. To assess improvement, look at your level of ease in jumping this distance repeatedly — is it challenging, can you always do it, etc.

Broad Jump

With your feet shoulder-width apart, swing your arms and jump forward with both feet. Continue jumping in succession for 3-5 jumps. The timing of your arm swing can dramatically help with the distance of your jump.

Are you improving? Consider measuring how far your longest jump is, and try to break your record. Also, try jumping three times in a row, and measure the total distance. Compare your results after a month to see if you're jumping further.

One Foot Balance

Good balance is often associated with agility. Try improving your balance simply by standing on one foot. See how long you can balance. Try your luck on each legs.

Figure 8 Pattern

At a brisk walk, or jog, follow a large Figure 8 pattern, for 3-5 minutes. Then, change directions and complete the Figure 8 in the other direction. With practise, decrease the size of the Figure 8 and increase your time completing the exercise.

Lifestyle activities which encourage agility:
soccer, football, tennis, badminton, basketball.

Flexibility

This is a key component in overall fitness, yet many lose their flexibility as they get older. So when you're young it's great to maintain and/or improve what you have, to help set the stage for later in life. If you're only considering this, or noticing a decline in flexibility later in life, there is still many ways to improve your level of flexibility now.

Repetition and consistency are crucial — being flexible isn't something you achieve after two weeks; it takes time and regular effort. Also, this term can apply to a range of different areas of your body — it isn't as easy as a simple "Can I touch my toes?"

KEY POINTS: Always start slow and always hold the stretch. Don't bounce. It's easier on your muscles if you're "warmed up" prior to stretching, so increase your heart rate slightly by lightly running or fast walking on the spot before beginning.

Additionally, pain is not a good sign. When stretching, lean into a stretch until you can feel it; then hold it, ideally for 10-20 seconds. Release your stretch and relax for 30 seconds; stretch again and hold.

As a result, you should gain suppleness and the ability to achieve a full range of movements — turning, twisting and bending — without any stiffness or aching.

Toe Touch

Target area: Lower back, and back of your legs

Standing from the waist, bend over slowly, letting your body hang naturally. Then, with straight legs, reach towards the floor. When you've reached as low as you can go, gently hold that part of your legs with your dangling hands. If you can reach the floor, touch it instead, and hold. Release and return to where your body hung over naturally, and repeat. When you straighten up, be sure to bend your knees initially, and slowly curl your back to the upright position.

VARIATION: If standing isn't working for you, try doing this stretch while seated on the floor. Place your back against a wall, legs outstretched flat in front of you, and lean forward, to feel the stretch, reaching for your toes.

Are you improving? With repetition, over time, you should gradually be able to reach further and further down, or if you can touch the floor with only the tips of your fingers, then aim to touch the floor with the palms of your hands.

Chest Lift

Target Area: Back, chest

Lie flat on your stomach, with your arms behind your back. Slowly and gently lift your chin, shoulders and chest off the floor, while keeping your hips and legs lying flat. Hold 10 seconds, if possible, and lower your chest, shoulders and head back down. Then repeat the stretch 3-5 times. Be careful not to strain your neck with any twisting or rotation.

VARIATION: If it's more comfortable, try the exercise with your hands by your side.

Are you improving? Over time you should notice that you can stretch further up, raising more and more of your torso off the floor. If at the moment you can only lift your chin and part of your shoulders, then in the future you may be able to raise the top of your chest off the floor.

Shoulder Roll

Target Area: Shoulders, back

This is a simple yet effective exercise and stretch. Often flexibility is about restoring movement and loosening those muscles that were once supple and had a full range of motion.

While standing, or seated at a firm chair, bring your shoulders up to your ears and slowly roll them backwards in a circular motion, stopping momentarily in quarters around the circle (i.e., at positions 12, 3, 6, and 9 on a clock). Push your shoulders as low as they can go at the bottom of the circle, then bring them to the front and back up. Repeat this slow circle 5-10 times and then rest. Repeat in the opposite direction 5-10 times.

VARIATION: Once limber, try swinging your arms, fully extended, one at a time, in the same circular motion. It's important to be in control of your rotating arm instead of letting it swing freely, as that could result in injury.

Are you improving? With practise you should find this exercise easier to do. Your shoulders and upper body will be able to move in a larger "circle," and with less internal resistance.

Knee Hug

Target Area: Hips and buttocks

Lie on your back, with your legs outstretched and arms at your side. Slowly bring up one leg, bent at the knee, towards your chest. Wrap your arms around this bended leg, with your hands meeting below the knee. The goal is to keep the other leg, still on the floor, straight and in line with your hip. However, to begin with, your straight leg may want to come off the floor, and/or it may be difficult to "hug" your knee. Do this stretch 3-5 times, and repeat with the other leg.

VARIATION: If this exercise is difficult for you, try isolating the "hug" element. Lying flat on the floor, slowly bring both sknees towards your chest, grasping both legs with your hands; you should resemble a ball. Hold this stretch, breathing deeply, and release. Then repeat.

Are you improving? Over time, you should notice the bended knee pull in further towards your chest with greater ease and less internal resistance. Also, the straight leg should eventually feel comfortable at rest on the floor, instead of wanting to pull up.

Side Stretch

Target Area: Abdominals, arms

Stand upright, feet shoulder width apart. Reach your right arm slowly over your head and bend to the left slightly in the waist; your raised arm should be reaching overhead to the left as well. Your left arm stays at rest. You should feel a stretch under your arm and down the exposed side of your body. Hold this stretch, and then straighten up. Repeat 3-5 times and then try the stretch on the other side.

VARIATION: Try reaching upwards with your raised arm instead of letting it follow your abdominal bend — you should feel a lengthening stretch as well. Or, spread your feet apart greater than shoulder width and try the stretch from this position.

Are you improving? You should notice with time that your body can bend further, and deeper to the side.

Lifestyle activities which encourage flexibility:
yoga, tai chi, dance/ballet, stretching.

Cardiovascular

Cardiovascular refers to both the heart and lung components of fitness. It is the cornerstone of overall health and wellbeing. A well-tuned cardio system usually results in improvements across your whole body. The basic idea is to get involved in an activity which raises your heart rate and breathing to an elevated level, for an extended period of time, ideally for 20-40 minutes, depending on your fitness level.

However, you do need to monitor your heart rate to ensure it stays within a healthy range, and that you're not overworking yourself.

In regards to your breathing, here's the rule of thumb: you should always be able to carry on a conversation with a friend; if you're too winded to do this, you're working too hard.

When beginning a new cardio program, the key is to build up to the 20-40 minutes. If you haven't done any activity for a while, don't make your first workouts too long or you'll never want to work out again. For example, try 10 minutes for the first week; then add 5 additional minutes every week until you build up to your target of 20-40 minutes. Also, be sure to warm up, to get your heart rate going, before every session.

Jumping Rope

Get a skipping rope and find a wide area to jump in. Skipping is a very difficult exercise to do for prolonged periods. So, start slow; don't jump as fast as you can right away, but instead jump at a rate that you can hopefully sustain for several minutes.

VARIATION: Try alternating your jumping style: try on one foot, alternating feet; try jumping with your feet apart; or even try bringing your knees up high when you jump. Also, try varying the intensity: jump as fast as you can for 1 minute, and then at your regular speed for 5, repeating this pattern throughout your workout.

Are you improving? Measure your success by the length of time skipping, and the intensity/speed of your jumping. Both have their advantages and signal your ongoing improvement.

Swimming

Head to the local swimming pool, or perhaps just outside if you have your own pool, and swim a couple laps. With swimming, you're trying to maintain your increased heart rate, so swimming laps are an ideal activity.

VARIATION: You can use any stroke you like, or any combination or variation, but keep at it, and you can swim like you're Michael Phelps. Note: if you're not swimming in a life-guarded area, never swim alone.

Are you improving? Look for an increase in distance, or an ability to swim for a longer period of time. If time is limited, then try to swim harder than you were before, i.e., swimming a longer distance in the same amount of time.

Fast Walking

Grab a sturdy pair of walking shoes or gym shoes, and head outside. You don't need any equipment other than healthy determination to start walking. Though to help improve your cardio, you need to walk fast enough to get your heart rate up, so pick up the pace — this isn't a leisurely stroll. In bad weather, try the mall for a dry, covered area to walk.

VARIATION: Try alternating fast walking with light jogging. For example, try a combination such as walking 4 minutes, jogging 1 minute, for the duration of your workout. Or consider varying your route to include a hill or incline. Also, terrain makes a difference — walking on sand provides more resistance, while walking in the woods demands more thought and attention.

Are you improving? Over time, you should be able to walk faster, and for a longer period of time, without adding an uncomfortable amount of stress on your body. You can measure your improvement in terms of distance walked, steps taken, or distances that you walked in a certain amount of time. A pedometer will definitely help keep track of some of these figures.

Squash/Tennis

Racquet sports can be a great way to improve your cardio in a social setting. Get a fitness buddy and join a squash club. Squash is a great racquet sport that involves both coordination and cardio. Alternatively, if you've previously enjoyed tennis, try picking the sport up again.

VARIATION: You can also practice a sport like squash on your own, so try to challenge yourself and see how hard you can work out.

Are you improving? In sqaush or tennis, with improved skill you should notice longer rallies of play. It is in these longer rallies that you will notice your improvement — you should be able to keep the play going, and not stop due to fatigue. Provided you're not playing one of the Williams sisters . . .

Walking Stairs

This is the idea behind the trusty StairMaster, but the authentic version. Head up the stairs in your house, the local sporting arena, or any nearby flight of steps. Then, it's as easy as climbing up and down for a set amount of time. While climbing up definitely uses more energy and is more of a cardio workout, climbing down also requires effort from your system.

VARIATION: Once you've mastered this, try adding weight such as wrist weights or even carrying two bottles of water, to increase the amount of weight your body has to carry up the stairs.

Are you improving? Look for signs like climbing faster, breathing easier, and being able to climb for longer.

*Lifestyle activities which encourage cardio development:
cycling, running/jogging, boxing, soccer, dancing vigorously,
trampoline jumping, gym activities (treadmill, elliptical,
as well as tennis and squash, of course).*

Endurance

Endurance training involves low to medium-intensity exercising for longer periods, such as jogging several miles, instead of sprinting once around the block.

Tips for building endurance:

▸ *Aim for longer, slower paced workouts*

When striving to build endurance, slow and steady wins the race. Once you've decided on the time goal, set an appropriate pace so that you're able to sustain your activity throughout the time period. Pace yourself — this is playing the long game.

▸ *Dedication goes a long way*

Ideally, try to work out several times a week, and build up to daily workouts. As endurance training doesn't have the same intensity as strength training, daily workouts are fine. However, don't try to do too much at once: start at 5 or 10 minutes, and work your way up to 30-40 minutes of activity.

▸ *Positive mental attitude*

A large part of endurance is your mental attitude. Making a commitment to follow a fitness routine requires a certain mental attitude; it is this same perseverance that is also required when you're almost at the end of your energy. This means that towards the end of your cycle, jog or swim, dig deep and keep going. Take it one step at a time, and you can do it.

▸ *Balanced workout*

Incorporate all the other elements of fitness — strength, flexibility, agility and cardio — as each of these will help you achieve your endurance goals.

Lifestyle Activities which encourage endurance:
Swimming, bicycling, walking briskly, tennis, volleyball, rowing, dancing, climbing stairs or hills, skiing, hiking, jogging.

ABCs of Vitamins, Minerals and Nutrition

When having surgery, you're under the care of a capable health care team, but once you leave, you need to do everything you can for yourself. Thus, this section will provide the general nutritional support and advice that is vital for consuming the nutrients that any body requires to function at its peak performance.

Naturally, we don't all necessarily stick to a strict dietary regime of carrots and celery; a hamburger or a tempting bowl of chicken wings are bound to creep into the picture. Yet, especially after surgery, it's important to give your body an added boost, so it can get back on track and repair itself.

Nutrition falls into six major nutrition groups: carbohydrates, proteins, fats, vitamins, minerals, and water. Read on to learn some of the ways you can build a good nutritional base to help pave your road to recovery.

There are a total of 13 vitamins, which are essentially organic compounds that are necessary for your body's normal metabolic functions. They constantly need to be replenished as we lose them every time we urinate. So, it's important to ensure a daily intake of the nutrients you need.

Here's a cheat sheet of vitamins and what they do:

Vitamin A

WHY YOU NEED IT: This vitamin helps you see in the dark and promotes a healthy immune system. This includes aiding the growth and development of cells, keeping your skin healthy, and promoting the formation and maintenance of healthy teeth, too.

WHERE YOU FIND IT: Vitamin A can be found in milk, eggs, liver, fortified cereals, carrots, sweet potatoes, pumpkin, cantaloupe, apricots, peaches, papayas, and mangos — the majority of your orange fruits and vegetables.

Vitamin B1

WHY YOU NEED IT: All B vitamins help to create energy by breaking down and metabolizing fats and carbohydrates. In addition, vitamin B1, also known as thiamin, helps to maintain the heart's functions, and the nervous, cardiovascular, and digestive systems.

WHERE YOU FIND IT: Oatmeal, brown rice, whole grain flour, asparagus, potatoes, oranges, pork, liver and eggs.

Vitamin B2

WHY YOU NEED IT: Vitamin B2 (or riboflavin) aids the body's antioxidants, to protect against free radicals.

WHERE YOU FIND IT: Milk, cheese, green leafy vegetables, liver, kidneys, and legumes.

Vitamin B3

WHY YOU NEED IT: Vitamin B3 aids antioxidants and plays a role in our digestive systems. Be aware that deficiency of B3 (or niacin) can cause the disease pellagra (a vitamin deficiency); while in mild cases, lack of B3 may slow the body's metabolism, causing intolerance to cold.

WHERE YOU FIND IT: Often in pill form.

Vitamin B4

WHY YOU NEED IT: Vitamin B4 (or adenine) produces energy along with the other B vitamins.

WHERE YOU FIND IT: In whole grains (breads and cereals), raw honey, bee pollen, royal jelly, and most fresh vegetables and fruits.

Vitamin B5

WHY YOU NEED IT: Vitamin B5 (or pantothenic acid) is also known as the anti-stress vitamin because of its support of the adrenal gland's release of cortisol. It also stimulates the immune system to produce antibodies.

WHERE YOU FIND IT: Beef, eggs, fresh vegetables, kidney, legumes, liver, mushrooms, nuts, pork, saltwater fish, whole rye flour, and whole wheat.

Vitamin B6

WHY YOU NEED IT: Vitamin B6 (or pyridoxine) is crucial for normal brain function.

WHERE YOU FIND IT: In a variety of foods, including potatoes, bananas, beans, seeds, nuts, red meat, poultry, fish, eggs, spinach, as well as added to some breakfast cereals.

Vitamin B9

WHY YOU NEED IT: Otherwise known as folate, this vitamin is important in DNA production, producing new cell bodies, and preventing changes that may lead to cancer. Particularly important for expectant moms.

WHERE YOU FIND IT: Spinach, turnip greens, lettuces, fortified cereal, and sunflower seeds.

Vitamin B12

WHY YOU NEED IT: Vitamin B12 (or cobalamin) helps make red blood cells and gives you energy, of course.

WHERE YOU FIND IT: Fish, red meat, poultry, milk, cheese, eggs, and fortified cereals.

Vitamin C

WHY YOU NEED IT: Vitamin C is essential for healthy bones, teeth and gums. It also helps in the healing of wounds, and plays a part in forming collagen.

WHERE YOU FIND IT: In red berries, kiwi, red and green bell peppers, tomatoes, broccoli, spinach, and orange and grapefruit juice.

Vitamin D

WHY YOU NEED IT: Vitamin D strengthens bones by aiding in the body's absorption of calcium.

WHERE YOU FIND IT: Uniquely, this vitamin is manufactured when your skin is exposed to sunlight. It is also found in egg yolks, fish oils, and fortified foods such as milk.

Vitamin E

WHY YOU NEED IT: An antioxidant, vitamin E helps protect cells from damage and keeps red blood cells healthy.

WHERE YOU FIND IT: Found in many foods, such as vegetable oils, nuts, avocados, wheat germ, whole grains, and green leafy vegetables.

Vitamin K

WHY YOU NEED IT: Regulating normal blood clotting, vitamin K is part of the synthesis process of several proteins that are necessary for coagulation and anticoagulation. Also, it prevents the hardening of arteries, so can reduce the occurrence of heart disease and failure.

WHERE YOU FIND IT: Found in green leafy vegetables, in particular the dark ones such as spinach and kale, as well as cabbage, cauliflower, broccoli, and sprouts, and fruits such as avocado and kiwi. Parsley is full of vitamin K.

Top Five Minerals

Unlike vitamins and other nutrients, minerals are inorganic compounds. Typically, a mineral is usually nothing more than a molecule, or a couple of molecules, of an element. They help maintain normal function of your nervous system, cellular reactions, structural and skeletal systems, and water balance in the body.

There are many minerals found within the human body, but there are at least 16 "essential" minerals. Here are our top five, in reverse order:

5. *Potassium*

WHY YOU NEED IT: Potassium is an electrolyte that works alongside another mineral, sodium, to regulate the body's water levels. A poor potassium/sodium balance ultimately can lead to dehydration and weakness.

WHERE YOU FIND IT: Potassium is commonly found in all balanced diets that include foods like orange juice, potatoes, bananas, avocados, tomatoes, broccoli, and apricots.

4. *Iron*

WHY YOU NEED IT: Iron is a constituent of hemoglobin, which is responsible for transporting oxygen around your body. Thus, with a healthy amount of iron in the body you can get more oxygen to your muscles, and you will recover much, much faster.

WHERE YOU FIND IT: Red meat, fish, poultry, lentils, beans, tofu, chickpeas, black-eyed peas, fortified bread and breakfast cereals. Iron in meat is more easily absorbed than iron in vegetables.

3. *Sodium*

WHY YOU NEED IT: The human requirement for sodium in the diet is about 500 mg per day. Yet, many people consume far more sodium than is needed, so this may be a case of balancing your intake of sodium to get just the right amount. Together with potassium, this electrolyte plays an important role in the body.

WHERE YOU FIND IT: Table salt.

2. Zinc

WHY YOU NEED IT: Zinc is necessary for sustaining all life. And it's critical for all phases of growth: without it, you are susceptible to numerous chronic diseases.

WHERE YOU FIND IT: In pill form, but also naturally occurring in oysters, beans, nuts, almonds, whole grains, pumpkin seeds, and sunflower seeds.

1. Calcium

WHY YOU NEED IT: Great for teeth and bone-building, calcium is also needed for healthy muscles, hearts and digestive systems.

WHERE YOU FIND IT: Dairy products, calcium-fortified foods, canned fish with bones (salmon, sardines), and green leafy vegetables.

Balanced Diet

Find a balance with vitamins and minerals — make sure your intake is just right so that you get enough, but not too much, of one alone. Some turn to nutritional supplements such as a multivitamin to guarantee the consumption of a sufficient quantity of selected nutrients. However, when mixing and matching supplements, there is a chance that you might overdose or underdose on certain vitamins and minerals, which is a recipe for disaster.

Too much of one mineral, for instance, could cause a functional imbalance of another, or even negative side effects. As an example, if you consume too much zinc, you can inadvertently lower your HDL levels (the "good" cholesterol).

At the end of the day, the secret to getting a well-balanced proportion of nutrients is eating a healthy diet. Strive to follow the "five-a-day" rule of five portions of fruit and vegetables. Whole-grain breads and cereals, low-fat poultry and meat, non-fried fish, and low-fat milk, cheese and yogurt are also key factors in a balanced diet. It sounds simple, because it is!

Protein Power

Illness and injury take a nutritional toll on the body. People who have had surgery need extra protein, calories, and other nutrients that support this repair and recovery.

Those who are well-nourished are likely to recover from illness, injury, and surgery better and more quickly than those who are poorly nourished. Medical research has shown time and again that people who are not well nourished take longer to recover, are more likely to have complications, and are more likely to be re-hospitalized.

Protein is especially important for healing. The body uses the amino acids in protein to build and repair body cells and tissues. Those who are undernourished may not have the nutritional resources — especially the protein — they need for the body's "extra" work of healing.

4 Tips for a Protein-Packed Day

Extra protein can be especially beneficial if you're embarking on a major healing process, such as during post-surgery recovery. These suggestions will help you get more protein and extra calories in about the same amount of food you usually eat.

1.   Add nonfat dry milk or powdered protein supplements to regular whole milk. You can also add them to sauces and gravies or use them for breading meat, fish, or poultry. Cook cereals with milk instead of water. Use milk, half and half, and evaporated milk when making instant cocoa, canned soups, mashed potatoes, and puddings. Add extra ice cream to milkshakes. One cup of whole or nonfat milk contains about eight grams of protein.

2.   Add small pieces of meat, fish, or poultry to soups and to vegetable, noodle, and rice casseroles. A three-ounce portion of meat, fish, or poultry contains approximately 21 grams of protein.

3. Add grated cheese to cream sauces, casseroles, or vegetables. Melt sliced cheese over hot apple pie. Combine cottage cheese and cream cheese with fruit. Use cream cheese and margarine on hot bread or rolls. A one-ounce slice of American cheese contains about 5 grams of protein. One-half cup of cottage cheese has approximately 12 grams of protein.

4. Blend finely chopped hard-boiled eggs into sauces, gravies, chopped meats, or salad dressings, or sprinkle over salads. One very large egg contains about 6 grams of protein.

Ultimately, changing to a healthier lifestyle is key to getting better after surgery and onwards for the rest of your life, leading to increased wellness and longevity, as well as peak physical fitness.

Eating the right things and exercising regularly isn't a big secret. But, the real secret to success is finding your passions: the foods that taste great, and deliver vitamins, proteins and minerals; and the lifestyle exercises that you enjoy, like playing tennis, golf, or squash, or going swimming and jogging with a friend. Only then will you give your body what it needs, while putting a smile on your face.

It's our job to give our patients a winning smile. The next steps of keeping that smile are the choices you make.

Good luck and thanks for reading!

NOTES

NOTES

NOTES

NOTES

NOTES

NOTES